NUTRITION-BASED HEALTH

Nutricines and Nutrients, Health Maintenance and Disease Avoidance in Animals

NUTRITION-BASED HEALTH

Nutricines and Nutrients, Health Maintenance and Disease Avoidance in Animals

Clifford A Adams

NOTTINGHAM
University Press

Nottingham University Press
Manor Farm, Main Street, Thrumpton
Nottingham, NG11 0AX, United Kingdom

NOTTINGHAM

First published 2007

British Library Cataloguing in Publication Data
Nutrition-based Health: Nutricines and Nutrients, Health Maintenance and Disease Avoidance in Animals
Adams, CA

ISBN 978-1-904761-58-7

Typeset by Nottingham University Press, Nottingham
Printed and bound by Hobbs the Printers, Hampshire, England

CONTENTS

Preface

The care and raising of animals for food production is now a very large and important activity on a global basis. It supplies large volumes of high quality, low cost food for the human population. There is also an important international trade in food from animals which gives the animal production industry a significant economic value.

However the successful maintenance and development of the animal production industry will depend upon the ability to manage animal health. Good animal health is an important parameter for the efficient production of large volumes of low cost food and is important to minimize the risk of zoonoses where animals can pass on diseases to humans. Animal health also has major national and international economic consequences as disease outbreaks consume public sector resources and seriously disrupt international trade.

It is obviously important for both producers and consumers, that large volumes of low cost food are produced from healthy animals. However it is also evident that consumers and legislative authorities do not want those animals treated with drugs and medicines in order to keep them healthy. This inevitably leads to an increased focus upon nutrition as a means to maintain health and to avoid disease which is an ideal scenario for the production of food of animal origin.

It is important that those engaged in raising of animals for food appreciate and respond to these various concerns. This was the impetus for my first book ; « NUTRICINES Food Components in Health and Nutrition. » Here I attempted to show that that are many natural components of feed and food, the nutricines, that have valuable and beneficial effects in relating health to nutrition.

The second book, TOTAL NUTRITION, was an attempt to develop further the use of nutrients and nutricines in animal nutrition. The objective in Total Nutrition is to obtain the maximum value of various nutrients and nutricines at all stages of the animal production chain from feed raw materials to the nutrition of the mature animal.

In this third book, the focus is solely on NUTRITION-BASED HEALTH. Here a strategy of health maintenance and disease avoidance is further developed through the judicious application of nutricines and nutrients in animal feeds. The significance of feed components and animal health is discussed in Chapter 1. This is followed by the influence of feed on the genome and gene expression in Chapter 2. Chapter 3 deals with feed-pathogen interactions. Feed-mycotoxins interactions are presented in Chapter 4. Chapters 5, 6, and 7, deal with feed-host interactions. Gastrointestinal integrity is presented in Chapter 5, nutrition and the immune system is discussed in Chapter 6 and oxidative stress is addressed in Chapter 7. Feed intake and health assessment is covered in Chapter 8, and some general conclusions are offered in Chapter 9.

It is likely that nutritionists in the future will need to consider nutritional strategies for health maintenance and disease avoidance as important as nutritional strategies for zootechnical performance. The opposition to the use of drugs and medicines in animal production as manifested by the complete ban on antibiotic growth promoters in the EU in 2006 leads to an increased focus upon nutrition. It is challenging but also exciting to realise that in the further development of modern animal production:

"NUTRITION IS ALL THERE IS"

Clifford A. Adams

1 Feed Components: Nutrients and Nutricines in Nutrition-based Health

The care and raising of animals for food production is now a very large and important activity on a global basis. It is the major occupation of 1.3 billion people worldwide and accounts for 40% of agricultural gross domestic product (Steinfeld *et al.*, 2006).

Foods of animal origin provide about one-sixth of human food energy consumed globally and one-third of the protein (Chadd *et al.*, 2002). They are energy-dense and an excellent source of high-quality and readily digestible protein. The proteins in these foods are the highest quality available for human nutrition as they contain a full complement of amino acids, and closely resemble the proteins of the human body in their amino acid composition. Proteins of animal origin by and large are more easily digested by humans than are proteins of plant origin and one hundred grams of lean meat provides up to half our daily protein requirement.

Meat is also an important source of various other nutrients in addition to amino acids, such as iron, selenium, zinc, vitamins A, B_{12} and folic acid. Some of these nutrients are either not present in food of plant origin or have a poor bioavailability. For example the vitamins A and B_{12} only occur in meat. Neither can be obtained from foods of plant origin. The carotenoid ß-carotene in plants is a putative provitamin A but needs to be consumed in high amounts due to a poor conversion rate in the body. Furthermore meat as a protein-rich food source is also carbohydrate-low and contributes to a low glycaemic index which is assumed to be beneficial in terms of non-infectious diseases such as obesity, diabetes and cancers (Neumann *et al.*, 2002; Biesalski, 2005).

Meat consumption has increased by, on average, more than 10% worldwide since the beginning of the 1960s. Average annual consumption per person has increased by more than 20kg during that period in Latin America, the Caribean, East Asia and the industrialized countries. The consumption of meat is highest, on average close to 90 kg/year in North America and most other industrialized countries (Valsta *et al.*, 2005). Recent projections have shown that world meat demand will continue to grow at a rate of 1.8% per year from 1993-2020. In 2000 global meat consumption was 233 million tonnes and is expected to rise to 300 million tonnes in 2020 and to 465 million tonnes in 2050. Milk production will rise from 568 to 700 million tonnes in 2020 and to 1043 million tonnes in 2050. Egg production will also increase by 30% (Speedy, 2002; Steinfeld *et al.*, 2006).

Good animal health is clearly an important parameter for the efficient production of the large volumes of food of animal origin which are currently required, and the even greater volumes which will be required in the future. Animals in poor health will not be as productive as healthy animals and consequently will yield lower volumes of food products for the human population. Therefore health maintenance and disease avoidance in the animals raised for food in modern animal production is a major global challenge. Animal health impacts greatly upon the security of an important food supply, upon human health and upon international economics.

The status of animal health is also important to minimize the risk of zoonoses, where animals can pass on diseases to humans. Dairy cattle for example can pass on tuberculosis to humans but this has largely been controlled. Also the possible association of Johne's disease in cattle with Crohn's disease in humans and bovine spongiform encephalopathy (BSE) with variant Creuztfeld-Jacob disease in humans are important concerns. Avian influenza is also a zoonotic disease but fortunately at this time transmission to humans does not readily occur. Micro-organisms such as *Salmonella* in pigs and *Campylobacter* in broilers are not in themselves pathogens for the host animal, but they may readily contaminate meat obtained from these animals and subsequently cause diseases in humans. In the EU *Campylobacter* has been recognised as one of the public health priorities among the food borne zoonotic pathogens (Anon, 2004).

The status of animal health nowadays has major national and international economic consequences. Diseases such as BSE, Foot and Mouth disease and Avian influenza are economically disastrous for the global animal production industry. They result in the mass culling of millions of animals which consumes public sector resources and seriously disrupts international trade. Frequently the outbreak of a serious animal disease on one country is followed by other countries instituting bans on exports of food of animal origin from the affected country. Therefore health maintenance and disease avoidance in animals raised for food is extremely important.

Health maintenance and disease avoidance

Health problems will have many possible origins and will require multiple solutions. Maintenance of health against a disease challenge can be considered as comprising two components; resistance and resilience (Klasing, 1998). Resistance refers to the ability of various protective systems such as skin and the immune system to exclude and remove pathogens from the body so that they cannot cause disease. Resilience refers to the ability of an animal to maintain productivity during an infectious challenge. This means that infected animals can continue to grow and show good productive efficiency. It is highly likely that diets designed to optimise resistance may not be optimum to support resilience and good productivity.

Some of problems of health maintenance and disease avoidance in animals are undoubtedly related to the demands of a modern society for large volumes of food of animal origin. This requires intensive animal production, raising large numbers of animals in relatively small areas. The combination of large numbers of animals with high productivity inevitably means that animals are exposed to considerable stress during their productive period. Stress, which arises from exposure of the animal to external forces and conditions, disturbs the homeostasis of the body and leads to the development of various pathologies. Examples of stress pathologies would be the transmission of infectious diseases due to micro-organisms, or the development of many non-infectious diseases due to environment or diet. These will have an important influence upon health maintenance and disease avoidance in animals.

The external forces and conditions that give rise to stresses in modern animal production have several origins. The raising of large numbers of animals in small areas increases the microbial stress on the animals. There is an increased risk of the rapid transmission of infectious organisms such as rotavirus, *Escherichia coli, Salmonella* species, *Clostridia perfringens* and *Campylobacter* species among animal populations. The time immediately after hatching or birth is a period of stress for most animals. The gastrointestinal tract of new-born animals is immature and sterile and begins to develop its function and its microflora when it begins to ingest feed. At this time the animal is very susceptible to pathogenic micro-organisms as the animal usually has little or no natural defences. In mammals, particularly calves and piglets, weaning imposes a severe stress when they are frequently moved to another location and receive a new and completely different diet than the milk-based diet they obtained from the mother.

Extensive preventive medication and vaccination is also a major contributor to stress.

There is a whole host of non-infectious diseases such as ascites in poultry, cardiac problems and joint and leg problems in many species. Non-infectious disease have a set of initiating factors that activate specific patterns of gene expression that in turn act to tip biochemical equilibria to non-homeostatic states. If prolonged, these non-homeostatic states produce tissue degeneration and loss of function of one or more organs and ultimately produce signs and symptoms that lead to a clinical diagnosis of disease. Gene expression studies are beginning to show differential expression of sets of genes in tissues from non-infectious diseases as compared to healthy tissue (Kornman, *et al.*, 2004). A non-infectious disease only develops if there is an altered expression of a specific set of genes. This altered pattern of gene expression may be the result of a combination of factors such as environment, genetic origin and nutrition.

The health status of animals may also be related to the genetic selection of food animals for superior growth and productivity that has occurred over the last 50 years. Many successful breeding programmes have led to the introduction of pig and poultry genotypes capable of rapid growth rates and lean muscle deposition coupled with high reproductive performance. For example, over the years 1989-96 the body weights of broilers increased from 1.80–2.25 kg whilst during the same period the FCR dropped from 1.984-1.843 (Cobb, 1999). There were further improvements in broiler performance in the USA over the years 1997-2001 (Chapman *et al.*, 2003). In this period there was a linear decrease in calorie conversion of the broilers. This is the feed conversion ratio multiplied by the average feed energy and is an index of the efficiency of feed utilization. The number of days to produce a 2.27 kg bird dropped from 49.5 days in 1997 to 46.5 days in 2001. Final body weight also increased from 2.22 kg to 2.35 kg. These are huge improvements in growth rate since over a five year period the growing time was reduced by 6.1% and yet final bird weight was increased by 5.8%. Data on laying hens collected over the years 1972-1996 show there has been a very significant improvement in feed utilization and egg production (Flock, 1998). In 1996 it was possible to produce one kilo of eggs with about 500 g less feed than was required in 1972.

There is some concern that this successful selection for improved productivity may be coincidentally associated with decreased resistance to disease or changes in immunological response (Cheema *et al.*, 2003; Li *et al.*, 2001). In pigs there is a concern about high mortality in both weaned pigs and sows. Longevity of sows in a sow herd is of major concern in many commercial pig herds. The highest producing and fastest growing animals, both pigs and poultry, may suffer heavy mortalities due to sudden deaths

This problem is illustrated in a study with commercial turkeys comparing a fast growing heavy line with a slow growing medium line from the same breeder (Kowalsksi *et al.*, 2002). The fast growing line was more sensitive to adverse environmental factors and had a much larger increase in corticosterone when exposed to transport stress than the slow growing line. The slow growing line showed more adaptability to stress. Further work with turkeys showed that a response to stress was altered by selection for increased body weight (Huff *et al.*, 2006). This may make the turkeys more sensitive to chronic bacterial diseases such as turkey osteomyelitis complex. There is clearly a need to develop nutritional and environmental strategies to modulate the stress response pathologies in modern animals raised for food production.

Feed is also a potential source of stress. Clearly adequate levels of nutrients to support the rapid growth rates and high productivity must be supplied to animals through feed. However feed must inevitably be produced as cheaply as possible from available raw materials to maintain the economic viability of modern animal production. Feed ingredients such as wheat, barley and fats are known to cause digestive stress in some species. Feed inevitably contains micro-organisms and other components which may be toxic and puts additional stress on the animal, either through diseases or activation of the immune system.

Health management

Although animal health is clearly a major concern in modern animal production, in reality, there are few options to manage animal health. Diseases such as necrotic enteritis in poultry and histomoniasis in turkeys were controlled in the recent past through various pharmaceutical products but most of these have now been banned in the EU and no alternative products are available. There is a considerable range of effective vaccines for some diseases but vaccination is not a suitable response for many devastating diseases such as Avian influenza, BSE or PMWS (post-weaning multisystemic wasting disease in pigs). For these reasons mass culling programmes are frequently instituted to control animal diseases.

Furthermore there has been a significant shift in consumer and legislative attitudes in the EU and elsewhere towards treating animals raised for food with pharmaceutical products. In general consumers want food from healthy animals but they do not want animals treated with drugs and medicines. This is well exemplified by the complete ban on antibiotic growth promoters which came into force in the EU in 2006.

The inability to mount effective large scale therapeutic programmes to control diseases in animals requires a major paradigm shift from the treatment of clinical illness to health maintenance and disease avoidance. The emphasis now must be on reduction of the various stress factors which predispose animals to disease. Therefore nutritional strategies to alleviate or avoid stress on the animals must be introduced in a Nutrition-based Health (NbH) approach. Such nutritional strategies however must be conducted in an economically viable manner which also recognises animal welfare, food safety, public health and environmental sustainability as illustrated in Figure 1.

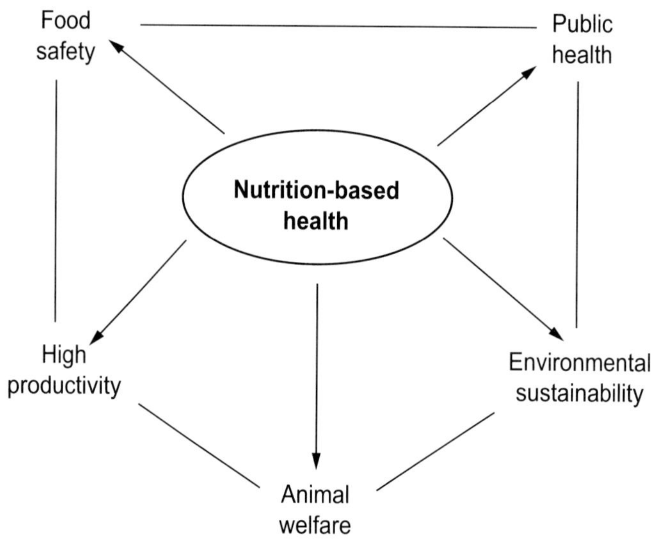

Figure 1. Interactions of nutrition-based health.

This focuses attention upon nutrition as the only practical solution to maintain animal health and to avoid disease and this is also very much in line with modern trends in human nutrition where diet and health interactions are increasingly investigated and promoted. There is a clear movement towards linking agriculture and nutrition with the major objective of developing health maintenance and disease avoidance strategies in humans (Schneeman, 2000). This will require some radical re-thinking to understand and take advantage of nutrition and health interactions in animal production (Adams, 2006).

The fundamental basis of nutrition is that all animals, including humans, have a continuous need to ingest complex mixtures of many different molecules in the form of feed or food. These various dietary components exert a multitude of activities and functions. These may be beneficial in supporting development, growth, health maintenance, and disease avoidance. Other feed components such as mycotoxins and microbial pathogens may be deleterious in generating non-infectious and infectious diseases.

The portfolio of materials ingested as feed is extremely diverse because over evolutionary time various animal species have developed different nutritional strategies varying from carnivorous to vegetarian. These strategies require different dietary materials and consequently the hosts are exposed to different amounts and types of feed-derived molecules.

This variation in dietary habits is associated with a particular digestive physiology. For example true carnivores such as the cats have a simpler digestive system than humans because animal products generally do not require prolonged digestion times. At the other end of the scale plant-eaters such as cattle and horses consume a large amount of cellulose which is not easy to digest but which they must use as an energy source. Vegetarian animals have evolved specially enlarged parts of the digestive tract to digest this cellulose by fermentation. This is the function of the rumen in cattle and the caecum and colon in horses. The human gastrointestinal tract however does not fit neatly into either of these two extreme categories which reflects our omnivorous or diverse dietary habit. Humans occupy an intermediate position as omnivorous, eating an extremely wide range of materials from both animal and plant origin, which also exposes them to the complete range of nutritionally-derived molecules available on this planet.

Nutrition-based Health (NbH), the application of feed components in health maintenance and disease avoidance must be based upon sound scientific principles and there are certainly difficulties in studying the relationship between diet, and disease development and control in animals.

This illustrates a major contrast between pharmacology and nutrition, even though pharmacology has frequently served as a model for nutritional research. The widespread use of antibiotics in animal nutrition has tied pharmacology and animal nutrition even closer together. However in the search for pharmaceutical molecules to cure or eliminate a particular disease there is a recognised disease state which is used as the research target. Therapeutically active molecules can then be discovered which will return the sick individual to a healthy one.

Such a programme cannot be adapted to a NbH strategy because the starting position is that of a healthy population of animals and the objective is to maintain that state of health. From this viewpoint all metabolic pathways in the animal's body must be performing optimally and the objective is to maintain this state. Conversely in the diseased state at least one pathway is not performing optimally and a pharmaceutical product will be used to rectify this and return it to a healthy condition.

Nutrition-based Health has more complexity than a pharmacological strategy as illustrated in the NbH triad (Figure 2), (Adams, 2006; Levander, 1997). This indicates that interactions between feed, pathogens and host characteristics all play a crucial role in determining the overall health and welfare status of animals.

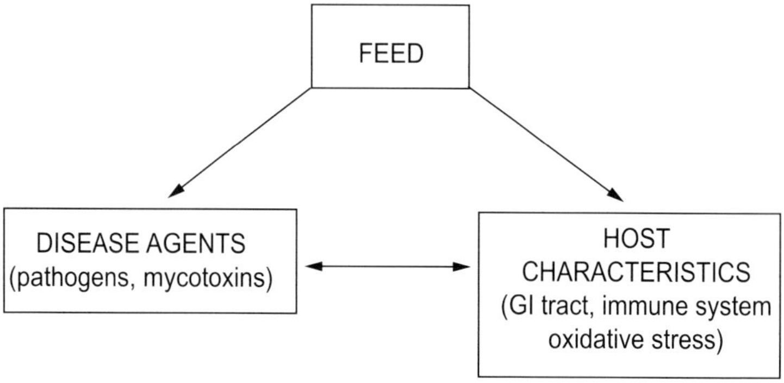

Figure 2. Nutrition-based Health triad.

The nature of feed therefore plays multiple roles in NbH through influencing the ability of the host to resist pathogens, by modulating the virulence of pathogens and by modulating non-infectious diseases. In particular nutrition has a great impact upon enteric diseases through modulation of the microflora in the gastrointestinal tract. Consequently managing the NbH triad (Figure 2) is an increasingly important research topic as animal health has to be protected and maintained through nutritional means.

The nature of feeds (nutrients and nutricines)

Modern animal nutrition is currently based upon feeds that are formulated using an array of available ingredients to supply a desired nutrient profile at the minimum cost. The practical nutritional characteristics of the feed are derived from previous research and field observations in order to avoid deficiency symptoms and to support the economically important production criterion of interest. This production criterion maybe; body weight, feed conversion efficiency, protein accretion, milk production or egg production, which could be expected from healthy animals.

Early work in nutritional science demonstrated that there were particular components in feed, the nutrients, which were important for growth and health and which needed to be supplied in suitable quantities. These include carbohydrates, fats, proteins, 17 mineral nutrients such as iron and iodine and 13 vitamins which may be either fat-soluble such as vitamin E or water soluble such as vitamin C. There are also nine essential amino acids which must be obtained from ingested proteins. A fundamental characteristic of nutrients is that they are continuously essential and a deficiency of nutrients rapidly translates into a deficiency disease.

Carbohydrates and fats are an important source of energy. Fats must also supply the essential fatty acids linoleic and linolenic as these cannot be produced in the animal body and the omega fatty acids are important constituents of nervous tissue. Plant foods are poor in omega fatty acids but they are quite common in animal fats and fish oils. An adequate supply of these fatty acids is particularly critical in early life when brain growth and development is underway.

Nutrients have many important functions, including supplying energy for cellular activity and they are a source of raw materials for the synthesis of new cellular structures. Many nutrients, particularly minerals and vitamins play a role in innumerable biochemical transformations in cells and may be considered to be involved in molecular nutrition, as opposed to supplying energy or raw materials for growth.

Feed however is not simply a collection of useful nutrients but in reality is a source of innumerable different molecules some of which may be toxic but many of which have important bioactivities. In recent years there has been increasing interest in those molecules in feed which are not classical nutrients yet have important biochemical functions or bioactivities at a cellular level. These feed components have been described as; nutricines (Adams, 1999), non-nutritive components (Roberfroid, 1999b), bioactive components (Klink, 2002) and food bioactives (Gillies, 2003). Whatever the terminology, there is clearly a recognition that feed components consist of at least two groups of molecules; NUTRIENTS and other bioactive components, NUTRICINES, which are not classical nutrients, as illustrated in Figure 3.

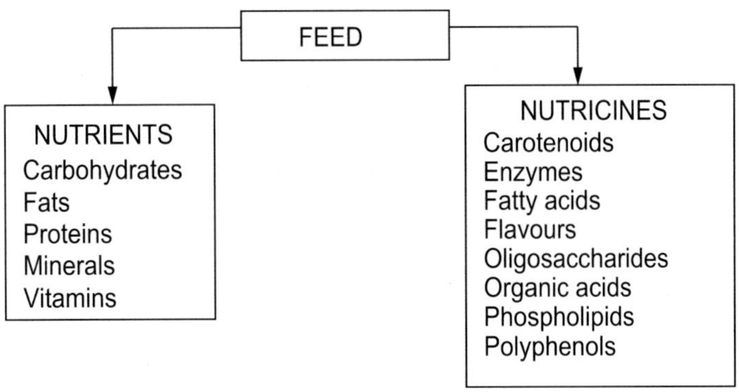

Figure 3. Components of food: nutrients and nutricines.

The nutricines play an important role in health maintenance and disease avoidance and the bioactivities of the nutricines are an important aspect of any NbH strategy.

Nutricines such as organic acids, phospholipids and various fatty acids are found in feedstuffs of both plant and animal origin. Polyphenols, carotenoids and oligosaccharides are primarily found in plant–based feedstuffs.

Obviously the groups of molecules comprising the nutrients and nutricines are not entirely exclusive to each group. For example fatty acids and organic acids can ultimately contribute to the energy supply of the cell and in this role they function as nutrients. However they also have several distinct biological activities not directly related to energy metabolism and here they clearly function as nutricines.

The necessity for the regular consumption of feed, exposes the cells and tissues of the animal to an enormous diversity of environmental inputs on an continuous basis. Feed consumption has always, and inevitably, been associated with the intake of a diverse range of nutricines as well as the essential nutrients. Nutricines have clearly been consumed by animals as long as nutrients have been consumed. Therefore it is hardly surprising that over evolutionary time this wide range of ingested nutricines in feeds would exert many effects upon the development and growth of the animal. These would be external effects in the gastrointestinal tract and internal effects at the cellular level.

Nutricines are quite polyvalent in their activities as illustrated in Table 1 and Figure 3 and can act at several different sites and levels in the body. They have several major types of bioactivities. They manage the gastrointestinal tract to avoid enteric diseases and help in the digestion and absorption of nutrients. This impacts upon nutrient availability. They offer protection against pathogenic micro-organisms through supporting the immune system and against non-infectious diseases by control of oxidative stress

Table 1. Various nutricines and their biological activities.

Major group	*Examples*	*Origin*	*Biological activity*
Carotenoids	Lutein, lycopene, capsanthin	Grass, tomatoes, spinach, paprika	Antioxidant, immunomodulator
Flavonoids	Flavonols,	Vegetables	Antioxidants
	Flavanones	Citrus fruits	Immunomodulator
	Flavanols	Green tea	Antioxidants
Carbohydrates	Resistant starch	Cereals and peas	Increased butyrate in large intestine
	Non-digestible oligosaccharides	Chicory, soyabeans, artichokes,	Modify gut flora, modulate lipid metabolisms
Organic acids	Lactic, citric, fumaric	Fruits, whey by-products	Antimicrobial activities
Phospholipids	Lecithins, lysolecithins	Soyabeans, rapeseed	Nutrient absorption
Phytic acid	Inositol hexaphosphate	Cereals and soyabeans	Antioxidant
Tocopherols	Gamma- and delta-tocopherols	Vegetable oils	Antioxidant

The full role of nutrition in health will be based upon multiple interactions between nutricines, nutrients and the genome, at the level of DNA, RNA, protein and metabolites (Figure 4), (Roche, 2006). Also the nature and duration of nutrient and nutricine exposure throughout an animal's lifetime will have an important impact upon health maintenance and disease avoidance.

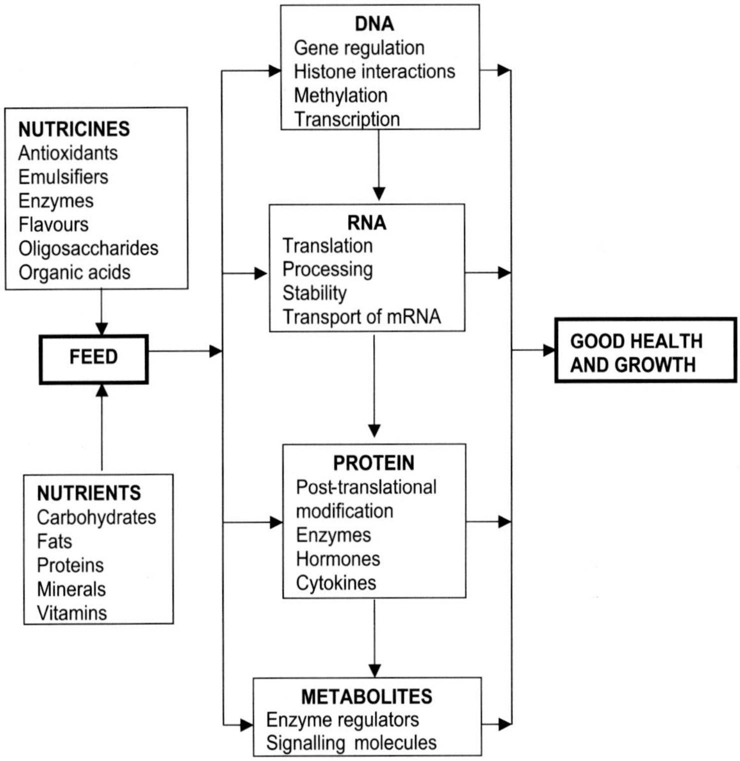

Figure 4. Nutrients and nutricines in feed interact with DNA, RNA, proteins and metabolites which influence growth and health.

Many nutricines act at the biochemical level, in the control of gene expression. Although the inherent genetic structure or genotype will have a considerable influence upon the structural architecture of the final phenotype, the nature and timing of environmental inputs is also extremely important. Regular environmental inputs such as the ingestion of nutricines in feed plays a major role in controlling both the expression of the genes in the genome and in determining the biological events necessary for the development and success of the phenotype. Feed can be seen as a source of environmental inputs with many different functions which play an important role in the gene/environment interaction that determine the phenotype of the organism.

At the simplest level nutrients and nutricines can have direct and immediate effects through up- or down-regulating genes and influencing subsequent protein expression. More complex time-dependent interactions also occur. For example early nutrition can induce epigenetic changes to the genome that have an impact upon diseases in adult life. This is manifested in problems of post-weaning stress in piglets. If piglets suffer serious post-weaning stress they never recover their full growth potential. Possibly a post-weaning stress induces some epigenetic changes which persist throughout the life of the pig.

An example of nutricines influencing gene expression is the observation that the plant-derived nutricines, curcumin and caffeic acid, are potent inducers of haem oxygenase enzymes through mediation of regulatory DNA sequences known as antioxidant-responsive elements (Balogun *et al.*, 2003). Haem oxygenase is a ubiquitous protein that protects cells against oxidative stress and it has an important role in degrading haem to CO, iron and biliverdin.

The positive functions of feed in terms of health maintenance and disease avoidance is also inevitably counteracted by a hostile environment which is largely inimical to good health. Animals must compete against a host of other living organisms on this planet which include plants, insects, fungi, bacteria and viruses, many of which are pathogenic. Many chemical components of the environment are toxic and in particular living organisms have to contend with the "Oxygen Paradox". The paradox is that whilst oxygen is essential for life, it is also toxic to life through various oxidation processes. Consequently animals have evolved a wide array of antioxidant molecules and strategies to deal with the potentially toxic effects of oxygen.

Nutritional and biochemical research has made tremendous progress in recent years so that we now have an increased understanding of the role the various feed-derived molecules may play at the molecular level. Feed components influence the immune status, pathogen virulence, proliferation of cells, DNA repair and modulate oxidative stress. All these factors have a profound impact upon health maintenance and disease avoidance and therefore it is important to elucidate the detailed functions of feed at the molecular level. Detailed and fundamental information relating to NbH has been published as Molecular Nutrition (Zempleni and Daniel, 2003) or Preventive Nutrition (Bendich and Deckelbaum, 2005).

It is important to emphasize that the criteria generally used to formulate animal feeds do not usually take into account the importance of nutrition in animal health, but rather focus on the productivity of healthy animals. It is implicitly assumed that the animals are healthy and that they will stay healthy during the production period. However harsh practical reality frequently demonstrates that this is not always the case and that animals do suffer from poor health and from disease.

To develop a positive NbH strategy, it is necessary to consider the origins and types of diseases, and attempt to find nutritional solutions to support health maintenance and disease avoidance (Adams, 2002), whilst recognising that it is unlikely that simple therapeutic nutritional solutions will be found which will cure disease in sick animals. Therefore the basic strategy of NbH has to be preventive and focussed upon health maintenance and disease avoidance. Fortunately this approach is very much in line with current consumer and legislative attitudes, where food of animal origin should be obtained from healthy animals, but the health of these animals should not be dependent upon treatment with an array of pharmaceutical products.

Nutricines and functional foods

The term "functional food" is generally restricted to human nutrition and originated in Japan in the 1980s when it was used to describe foods fortified with specific ingredients imparting certain health benefits (Hilliam, 1998). It has also been defined by Roberfroid (1999a) as foods that "should have a relevant effect on well-being, and health or result in a reduction in disease risk." Therefore the advantages offered by functional foods are generally related to health maintenance and disease avoidance rather than to therapeutic effects of foods. In this respect the term "functional foods" perhaps is preferable to the term "nutraceutical" which is also used, but which has a connotation of pharmaceutical and therapeutic effects.

The development of functional food science began by considering the physiological efficacies and potential health benefits of antioxidants, phytochemicals, digestion-resistant oligosaccharides, physiologically functional oligopeptides, etc, (Arai 2005). These may all be described as nutricines. It is obvious that nutricines are frequently the active principles in functional foods and the development of functional foods is a commercial manifestation of NbH applied to human nutrition. Animal feeds are not usually described as "functional feeds" even though they may well have many functional attributes similar to those found in functional foods. Nevertheless it may well be advantageous in terms of public perception to emphasize that in an NbH approach similar nutricines and nutrients are being utilized in animal nutrition as are used in functional foods for humans. In effect an NbH programme is the design and application of functional feeds for animals. This demonstrates a further coincidence between feed and food characteristics and properties, which is an important consumer issue nowadays.

External and internal functions of feed

In order to achieve rapid growth and development animals must continually ingest an extremely complex mixture of thousands of different molecules in the form of feed. This means that the body is continuously exposed to a wide range of different chemical entities which in turn will have various physiological effects. These effects of the ingestion of feed are expressed in two distinct physical spheres or locations. One is external, in the lumen of the gastrointestinal tract, which in fact is still outside the body. Feed components, after digestion then pass from the lumen of the gastrointestinal tract into the tissues of the body where they exert an internal effect, as depicted in Figure. 5. Various nutricines and nutrients play an important role in both External and Internal Nutrition.

The effect different feeds will have on the External or Internal Nutrition of an animal is complicated by the bioavailability of the various nutricines and nutrients. The total content of a component in a feed is not always sufficient information to indicate its nutritional quality. Frequently only a portion of any particular feed component may be digested and absorbed by the body and have an internal effect. However the complete feed mass will always have an external effect.

External functions of food (nutrition in the gastrointestinal tract)

The gastrointestinal tract is a very large and complex organ and represents an interface between the metabolism of the body and the environment. It provides an extensive surface area over which direct contact takes place between a wide array of nutrients, nutricines, micro-organisms and exogenous toxins. The intestinal epithelium or lining of the gastrointestinal tract must be maintained in a good physical state to prevent the bulk transport of pathogens into the body, but it must also be sufficiently thin to actively transport nutrients.

The gastrointestinal tract is also the largest endocrine gland in the body and produces at least 20 hormones, regulatory peptides and their receptors. It is the largest site of the immune system in the body and is the location for the majority of the lymphocytes and other immune cells in the gut-associated lymphoid tissue (GALT). The immune response and in particular the innate immune system is of major importance in disease avoidance and health maintenance in the gastrointestinal tract.

The gastrointestinal tract is not only a reservoir for ingested feed but also has a very complex microbial population. There is an enormous diversity of the micoflora in the gastrointestinal tract which has not been fully characterised. There may well be over 1000 different microbial strains as illustrated by the isolation of 1,230 partial 16S rRNA gene sequences from the gastrointestinal tract of broilers (Lu *et al.*, 2003). In general the microbial population in the gastrointestinal tract comprises about 150 trillion (150 million million) pathogenic and non-pathogenic organisms per kg body weight. One of the major challenges in modern nutrition is to manage this microflora for the benefit of the host and to avoid the onset of enteric diseases. This requires an understanding of the interactions of the various components in feeds with the microflora in the gastrointestinal tract.

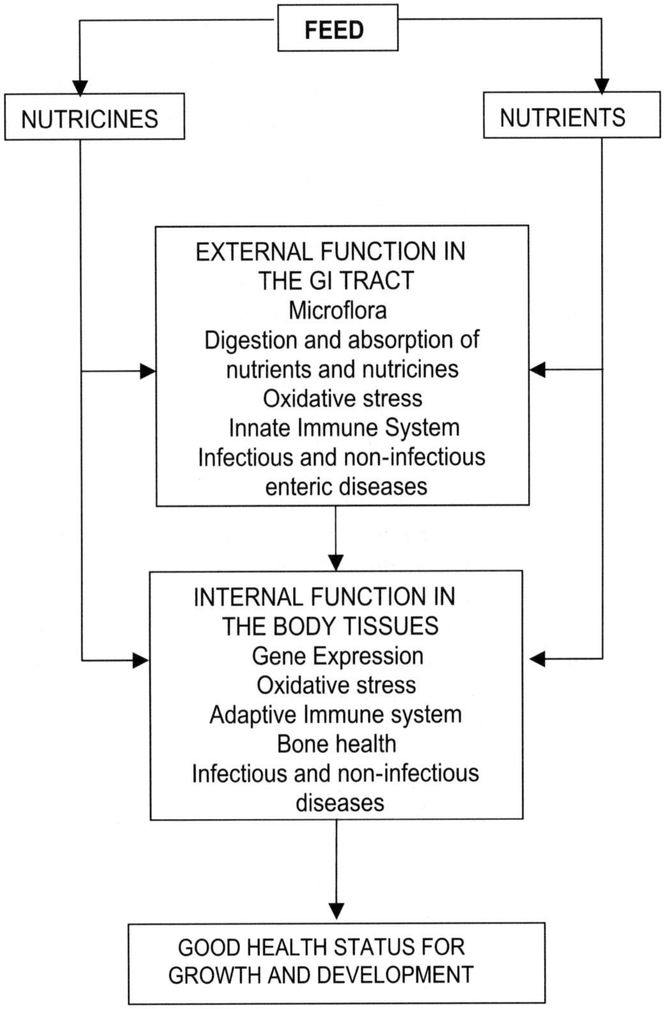

Figure 5. Nutricines and nutrients in external and internal nutrition.

Furthermore the gastrointestinal tract is expensive to maintain in terms of energy and protein requirements. It uses an enormous amount of nutrients for maintenance, tissue renewal and processing of nutrients. Any improvements to the health and efficiency of this organ would certainly lead to an overall improvement in the health and the development of the host. It is well recognised in animal production that various enteric diseases manifested as scouring or diarrhoea symptoms are a serious obstacle to efficient animal growth and performance.

A very important aspect of External Nutrition in the gastrointestinal tract is that it deals with a different spectrum of molecules than Internal Nutrition. Cells of the gastrointestinal tract are exposed to many large molecules such as dietary proteins, starch, cellulose, lignin, phytic acid and complex lipids. A large proportion of molecules such as proteins and starch will be digested into smaller units and then absorbed into the body of the organism where the constituent amino acids and glucose play a role in Internal Nutrition. There will be residual amounts of starch and protein that will not be digested and these will remain in the lumen of the gastrointestinal where they may be subjected to fermentation by the resident microflora. Other large molecules, which arrive in the gastrointestinal tract during ingestion of feed such as cellulose and lignins will not be digested at all in monogastric animals. A portion of these molecules may also be fermented in the large intestine into volatile fatty acids or they may pass completely through the gastrointestinal tract and be excreted in the faeces.

A major objective in External Nutritional is to manage the gastrointestinal tract so as to establish conditions which favour the growth of beneficial bacterial species such as *Lactobacilli* and *Bifidobacteria* which in turn will inhibit the growth of pathogenic organisms. This may be achieved by supplying non-digestible oligosaccharides, or fermentable carbohydrates (prebiotics) to encourage beneficial bacteria. Organic acid nutricines may play a useful role in the gastrointestinal tract as they are inhibitory to many pathogenic micro-organisms and butyric acid is also a useful energy source for cells of the large intestine. Protein degradation in the large intestine should be reduced and adequate glutamine supplied in the diet as an important energy source for the cells of the gastrointestinal tract.

Efficient digestion and absorption of feed depends initially upon the nature of the feed. There is an increasing tendency in the EU to manufacture animal feeds solely from plant-based raw materials. Many plant proteins however, are less readily digested than are animal proteins from meat and bone meals or fish meals. Increased use of cereals and oilseeds in animal feeds also increases the phytic acid content and the fibre content. Both phytic acid and dietary fibre are poorly digested by monogastric animals. Iron and calcium are poorly absorbed from plant sources (Neumann *et al.*, 2002). Some of these problems can be overcome by the use of supplemental feed enzymes to deal with phytic acid and fibre.

Absorption of digested feed materials also depends upon whether the digested components are in a suitable form (small units of peptides or of carbohydrates), whether the wall of the gastrointestinal tract is in a good healthy condition and whether there are inhibiting or promoting materials also present in the feed mixture. For example non-digestible oligosaccharides enhance calcium absorption from the gastrointestinal tract (Van Loo *et al.*, 1999; Scholz-Ahrens and Schrezenmeir, 2002). Obviously cells must be able to absorb sufficient quantities of the various nutrients and nutricines to satisfy their metabolic requirements in order to maintain good growth and development.

External Nutrition in the gastrointestinal tract has a very significant effect upon health and well-being of the host organism. It influences the microflora, digestive physiology, immune stimulation and inflammation. The gastrointestinal tract is the first site for infection by feed-borne pathogenic micro-organisms, and enteric diseases are a major health hazard for all animal species. Therefore an important function of feed in External Nutrition is to avoid enteric diseases and to promote good health and growth. Several nutricines such as enzymes, phospholipids, and organic acids play an important role in managing the gastrointestinal tract.

Internal functions of food (nutrition at the cellular level)

Internal Nutrition depends upon a supply of feed components from digestion and absorption of feed in the lumen of the gastrointestinal tract. The digestive process releases and solubilizes nutrients and nutricines so they can move out of the original feed matrix and diffuse or be transported to the cells of the wall of the gastrointestinal tract where they may exert various effects or they may be absorbed into the cells of the body where they subsequently influence gene expression and other metabolic activities. A major activity of Internal Nutrition is obviously supplying nutrients for energy metabolism and the biosynthesis of new cells and tissues for growth and development. This is the internal function of feed or nutrition at the cellular level. Much of the early work in nutrition establishing nutrient levels to avoid deficiency symptoms and to promote growth was in fact characterizing Internal Nutrition.

Various nutricines such as ß-glucans and carotenoids have recognised immunomodulating functions in cells (see Chapter 6). Development of an efficient adaptive immune system in the body is obviously an important contribution to health maintenance and disease avoidance.

It has now been demonstrated that a range of feed ingredients including carbohydrates, fatty acids, amino acids and carotenoids actively participate in the regulation of gene expression. Both nutrients and nutricines modulate the activity of transcription factors which are proteins that bind to specific DNA sequences within the promoter region of genes and can activate or inhibit their transcription. Feed components in Internal Nutrition play a dual role in modifying the phenotype of the animal. They provide the necessary energy sources and raw materials for development of the phenotype. Feed components, nutrients and nutricines, directly interact with the genotype and influence gene expression which will also modify the ultimate phenotype of the animal.

Conclusions

The care and raising of animals for food production is a very large and important global industry. Therefore health maintenance and disease avoidance in modern animal production is now a major challenge. It is important for food safety, to avoid zoonotic diseases being passed to humans, and also for efficient international trade.

Animals may be subject to considerable stress during the raising period which may be manifested as increased susceptibility to infectious diseases and the development of many non-infectious diseases. However the major route to maintain health and avoid disease must be through nutrition, and Nutrition-based Health (NbH) will become an important strategy in animal production. It also responds to consumer and legislative concerns where the link between diet and health is increasingly under investigation. Animal feeds however, are extremely complex containing both nutrients and bioactive components, the nutricines, and a NbH approach must utilize both groups of feed ingredients. Feed exerts both an external effect inside the gastrointestinal tract and an internal effect upon metabolism of the animal body. The NbH concept raises considerations of dietary recommendations since now the objective is not simply avoidance of deficiency diseases but health maintenance and disease avoidance. The important function of NbH is the ability to maintain health and to avoid disease in normal animals that are ostensibly healthy.

References

Adams C. A. (1999) NUTRICINES Food Components in Health and Nutrition, Nottingham University Press, Nottingham UK, 128 pp.

Adams C. A. (2002) TOTAL NUTRITION Feeding Animals for Health and Growth, Nottingham University Press, Nottingham UK, 244 pp.

Adams, C. A. (2006). Nutrition-based health in animal production. *Nutrition Research Reviews*, 19: 79-89.

Anon (2004). Opinion of the scientific panel on biological hazards on the request from the Commission related to *Campylobacter* in animals and foodstuffs. *The EFSA Journal*, 177: 1-10.

Arai, S. (2005). Functional food science. *Journal of the Science of Food and Agriculture*, 85: 1603-1605.

Balogun, E., Hoque, M., Gong, H., Killeen, E., Green, C. J., Foresti, R., Alam, J. and Motterlini, R. (2003). Curcumin activates the haem oxygenase-1 gene via regulation of Nrf2 and the antioxidant

–responsive element. *Biochemical Journal,* **371**: 887-895.

Bendich, A. and Deckelbaum, R. J. (2005). *Preventive nutrition. The comprehensive guide for health professionals.* Third Edition, Humana Press, New Jersey, USA 958pp.

Biesalski, H-K. (2005). Meat as a component of a healthy diet- are there any risks or benefits if meat is avoided in the diet ? *Meat Science,* **70**: 509-524.

Chadd, S. A., Davies, W. P. and Koivisto, J. M. (2002). Practical production of protein for food animals. In: *Protein Sources for the Animal Feed Industry.* Proceedings of an Expert Consultation and Workshop, held at Bangkok, Thailand. FAO, Rome pp.99-166..

Chapman, H. D., Johnson, Z. B. and McFarland, J. L. (2003). Improvements in the performance of commercial broilers in the USA: analysis for the years 1997-2001. *Poultry Science,* **82**: 50-53.

Cheema, M. A., Qureshi, M. A. and Havenstein, G. B. (2003). A comparison of the immune response of a 2001commecial broiler with a 1957 randombred broiler strain when fed representative 1957 and 2001 broiler diets. *Poultry Science,* **82**: 1519-1529.

COBB (1999). Commercial literature: Cobb 500 Maintaining the momentum

Flock, D. K. (1998). Genetic-economic aspects of feed efficiency in laying hens. *World's Poultry Science Journal,* **54**: 225-239.

Gillies, P. J. (2003). Nutrigenomics: the Rubicon of molecular nutrition. *Journal of the American Dietetic Association,* **103**: S50-55.

Hilliam, M. (1998). The market for functional foods. *International Dairy Journal,* **8**: 349-353.

Huff, G., Huff, W., Rath, N., Balog, J., Anthony, N. B. and Nestor, K. (2006). Stress-induced colibacillosis and turkey osteomyelitis complex in turkeys selected for increased body weight. *Poultry Science,* **85**: 266-272.

Klasing, K. C. (1998). Nutritional modulation of resistance to infectious diseases. *Poultry Science,* **77**: 1119-1125.

Klink, L. (2002). Milk-derived bioactives. *The World of Food Ingredients,* Sept. pp. 28-35.

Kornman, K. S., Martha, P. W. and Duff, G. W. (2004). Genetic variations and inflammation: a practical nutrigenomics opportunity. *Nutrition,* **20**: 44-49.

Kowalski, A., Mormede, P., Jakubowski, K. and Jedlinkska-Krakowska, M. (2002). Comparison of susceptibility to stress in two genetic lines of turkey broilers BUT-9 and Big-6. *Polish Journal of Veterinary Science,* **5**: 145-150.

Levander, O. A. (1997). Nutrition and newly emerging viral diseases: an overview. *Journal of Nutrition,* **127**: 948S-950S.

Li, Z., Nestor, K. E., Saif, Y. M., Anderson, J. W. and Patterson, R. A. (2001). Effect of selection for increased bodyweight in turkeys on lymphoid organ weights, phagocytosis, and antibody responses to fowl cholera and Newcastle disease inactivated vaccines. *Poultry Science*, **80**: 689-694.

Lu, J., Idris, U., Harmon, B., Hofacre, C., Maurer, J. L. and Lee, M. D. (2003). Diversity and succession of the intestinal bacterial community of the maturing broiler chicken. *Applied and Environmental Microbiology*, **69**: 6816-6824.

Neumann, C., Harris, D. H. and Rogers, L. M. (2002). Contribution of animal source foods in improving diet quality and function in children in the developing world. *Nutrition Research*, **22**: 193-220.

Roberfroid, M. B. (1999a). What is beneficial for health? The concept of functional food. *Food and Chemical Toxicology*, **37**: 1039-1041.

Roberfroid, M. B. (1999b). Concepts in functional food: the case of inulin and oligofructose. *Journal of Nutrition*, **129** (Suppl.) 1398S-1401S.

Roche, H. M. (2006). Nutrigenomics- new approaches for human nutrition research. *Journal of the Science of Food and Agriculture*, **86**: 1156-1163.

Schneeman, B. O. (2000). Linking agricultural production and human nutrition. *Journal of the Science of Food and Agriculture*, **81**: 3-9.

Scholz-Ahrens, K. E. and Schrezenmeir, J. (2002). Inulin, oligofructose and mineral metabolism-experimental data and mechanism. *British Journal of Nutrition*, **87**, Suppl. 2: S179-S186.

Speedy, A. W. (2002). Overview of world feed protein needs and supply. in: *Protein Sources for the Animal Feed Industry.* Proceedings of an Expert Consultation and Workshop, held at Bangkok, Thailand. FAO, Rome pp. 13-34.

Steinfeld, H., Gerber, P., Wassenaar, T., Castel, V., Rosales, M. and de Haan, C. (2006). Livestock's long shadow. Environmental issues and options. FAO, Rome, 390 pp.

Valstra, L. M., Tapanainen, H. and Männistö, S. (2005). Meat fats in nutrition. *Meat Science*, **70**: 525-530.

Van Loo, J., Cummings, J., Delzenne, N., Englyst, H., Franck, A., Hopkins, M., Kok, N., Macfarlane, G., Newton, D., Quigley, M., Roberfroid, M., van Vliet, T. and van den Heuvel, E. (1999). Functional food properties of non-digestible oligosaccharides: a consensus report from the ENDO project (DGX11 AIR11-CT94-1095). *British Journal of Nutrition*, **81**: 121-132.

Zempleni, J. and Daniel, H. (2003). Molecular Nutrition. CABI Publishing, Wallingford, UK, 423pp.

2 The Genome, Gene Expression and Feed

A fundamental activity in the growth and development of a living organism is management of the system of genes that is located in the genome. The development of an organism therefore involves temporal and organ-specific expression or suppression of networks of genes leading to the synthesis of specific proteins. The pattern of specific gene expression changes in response to external or environmental signals and this will lead to multiple outcomes, such as growth, differentiation, health maintenance, disease avoidance or disease onset and inhibition of growth. It is not surprising that over evolutionary time many bioactive dietary components, the nutricines, have been able to exert major effects in controlling expression of the genome. Dietary components comprise an important group of signals that enable a multicellular organism to co-ordinate its response to complex environmental changes and which in turn will influence growth and development. One of the challenges of Nutrition-based Health (NbH) is to understand the impact of dietary components upon gene expression and to ensure that appropriate nutrition is supplied to the animals to favourably influence gene expression.

The genome

The genome is the complete set of genes in an organism which are arranged on a finite number of pairs of chromosomes. All species have their own unique set of chromosomes, pigs have 19 pairs, cows 30 pairs, chickens 39 pairs and humans 23 pairs. The chromosomes are located in the nucleus of a cell which has long been recognised as the source of nearly all the DNA in a cell. The chromosomes are composed of chromatin, (Avramova, 2002) which is a combination of DNA and histone proteins. A typical eukaryotic cell contains as much as 2 m length of DNA if it were stretched end to end. Long lengths of DNA in eukaryotic cells must be stored in a compact and organized form so that enzymes can access DNA regions of high activity without causing the collapse of the rest of the structure. The DNA in the chromosomes must also be packaged and organized in a manner compatible with a number of nuclear events such as differential gene transcription, DNA replication, gene recombination and cell division.

The sequencing of the total genomic DNA in the chromosomes has revealed the number of genes in the genome of several organisms. The bacterium *Escherichia coli* has 4,290 genes, the fruit fly, *Drosophila* has 13,600 genes, the nematode worm *Caenorhabditis elegans* has 18,424 genes and both the mouse and human genomes are now estimated to contain around 30,000 genes and the rice plant may have up to 55,000 genes (Pennisi, 2005).

The linear polymers of DNA which make up the genes are organized and compacted into the nucleus with the aid of the histone proteins, which are basic and positively charged. The high level of sequence conservation among histones in different species indicates the primary importance of histones to the replication and regulatory processes. They interact with the acidic, negatively-charged DNA and form the highly ordered structural organization of chromatin. This results in coiling the long DNA molecule into a manageable form. Histone proteins can assemble into specific aggregates and this affords some control over accession of other proteins and molecules to the DNA itself.

Histone modification

In an active cell the chromatin must be decondensed to allow access to the DNA and promote gene expression and subsequent synthesis of mRNA. Conversely a very tightly associated and densely packed histone assembly would prevent access to that region of the DNA for both regulatory elements which would influence gene expression and transcription machinery which would initiate the production of mRNA

Consequently histones exhibit several forms of post-translational modification and this is also a major basis of the regulation of the DNA. In essence slight variations in histone sequence or post-translational modifications that reduce its positive charge such as acetylation or phosphorylation, affect their DNA binding ability. Transcription and replication activities become possible only when the histones are modified to release the DNA.

A range of histone acetyltransferase enzymes are therefore considered as transcriptional co-activators. These can acetylate specific lysines in histone proteins. Histone acetylation directs the local destabilization of repressive histone-DNA interactions. Targeted acetylation allows the basal transcriptional machinery to assemble a functional transcription complex. There are also histone deacetylases and these might provide a molecular mechanisms whereby transcription might be controlled continuously. The activity of histone deacetylase would be to return the DNA to the repressive configuration where transcription could no longer occur. The maintenance of gene activity would require the continued activity of the co-activators such as acetyltransferases. In this way transcriptional activity could be modulated continuously through variations in histone conformation. Histone acetyltransferases and deacetylases are now implicated in the fundamental mechanisms of transcription control.

Chemical modifications, including acetylation, methylation, phosphorylation, ubiquitinisation and ADP-ribosylation of the histone tails that protrude from the histone bundles around which DNA is wrapped within chromatin, have been described as histone decoration. The patterns of these decorations is believed to hold a histone code which might well play an important role in the activity of the genome (Strahl and Allis, 2000). Of particular interest is the recognition that dietary components can influence histone decoration. For example, the short chain fatty acid, butyric acid, is a promoter of histone acetylation in colonic epithelial cells in rats (Boffa *et al.*, 1992). The mode of action of butyric acid is actually as a potent inhibitor of histone deacetylase. Histone decoration is one of the ways in which the genome integrates exposure to both extrinsic and intrinsic signals, resulting in modulation of gene expression and thus alterations in phenotype. Deciphering the histone code and determination of how the code is manipulated by diet opens up the possibility of understanding the interaction of nutrition with the genome and implications for health.

DNA methylation

Whilst modification of histone proteins is one possible control system in the genome there is also modification of the DNA in the genome through methylation. Vertebrate DNA is primarily methylated on the base cytosine, in the dinucleotide CpG where cytosine precedes guanosine. DNA methylation involves the covalent addition of a methyl group to the 5-position of the cytosine ring to form methyl cytosine (Figure 1).

Figure 1. Cytosine and methyl cytosine.

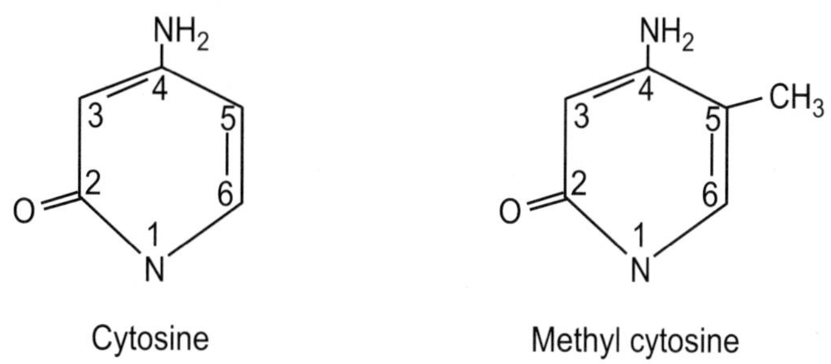

This is an epigenetic modification which occurs on approximately 5% of the cytosines in the mammalian genome (McCabe and Caudill, 2005). It is heritable but does not represent any change in the genetic information within the genome as there is no change in the primary base sequence, only the epigenetic addition of a methyl group.

Methylation is carried out by the action of DNA methyltransferase enzymes using S-adenolsylmethionine (SAM) as the methyl donor. The SAM in turn is generated through the methionine cycle.

DNA methylation has the ability to repress transcription and furthermore the patterns of methylation can be stably inherited during successive cell divisions. These two features make methylation very attractive as a potential regulator of gene expression during the development of an organism. It now well established that DNA methylation is an important regulator of gene activity in many organisms including vertebrates, fungi, and plants.

A general view is that DNA methylation acts as a global inhibitor of transcription due to the location of methylated cytosines throughout the genome thus preventing background transcriptional noise from the spontaneous activation of normally silent chromosomal regions. Moreover, DNA methylation is essential for normal vertebrate development and at least four mammalian cytosine DNA methyltransferases have been identified.

Aberrant DNA methylation has been associated with several disease conditions such as; birth defects, cancer, diabetes, heart disease and neurological disorders. For example human cancer cells often display abnormal patterns of low levels of DNA methylation or hypomethylation and this probably plays a causal role in tumour formation (Gaudet *et al.*, 2003; Eden *et al.*, 2003). Experimental mice mutants with abnormally low methylation in the genome were runted at birth and at four to eight months of age they developed aggressive tumours. It is likely that DNA hypomethylation plays a role in tumour formation by promoting chromosomal instability.

DNA methylation is influenced by drugs and dietary factors and has been shown to be reversible. This means that once the impact of dietary components on the DNA methylation is understood it should ultimately be possible to develop nutritional regimes that maintain the normal status of methylation patterns and which leads to good health.

Gene silencing which is related to methylation can be reversed by treatment with the DNA demethylating agent 5-aza-2′-deoxycytidine (azadC) (Lee and Chen, 2001). Several nutricines have also been shown to reverse DNA methylation and reactivate methylation-silenced genes. A gallic acid derivative from tea polyphenols (-) epigallocatechnin-3-gallate, and isoflavones from soyabean, particularly genistein, were able to re-activate genes silenced by methylation. The mechanism seems to be an inhibition of DNA methyltransferase activity by the nutricines (Fang *et al.*, 2003, 2005). This is epigenetic gene regulation and may contribute to the disease avoidance activity of various nutricines.

Several nutrients are also able to modulate DNA methylation; the most important being those supplying or regenerating methyl groups, which includes methionine, choline, folic acid, and vitamin B_{12}. Chronic deficiencies in nutrients which supply methyl groups will reduce DNA methylation. Generally in animal nutrition adequate levels of choline and methionine are formulated into feeds so deficiencies of methyl donors is unlikely. Nevertheless DNA methylation patterns may well be influenced by the nutritional status of the animal which would have consequent health effects. Also the possibility to actively modulate DNA methylation through a nutritional approach is an attractive research objective. The putative role of feed components both nutrients and nutricines interacting directly with DNA methylation patterns expands the whole concept of nutrition and NbH.

Epigenetics

Regulation of transcription of DNA enables cells to respond to environmental cues such as the availability of nutrients or viral infection. Consequently a failure to properly regulate transcription can lead to severe developmental abnormalities or to disease. One important regulatory process for DNA is through epigenetic changes. The main epigenetic features of the genome are DNA methylation and histone modification which alter gene expression without changing the DNA sequence. Epigenetic changes determine which genes are active and which are silent.

There is increasing evidence that aberrant DNA methylation and altered histone modification are features of ageing and of the development of many non-infectious diseases. Many dietary components are already known to influence epigenetic changes. For example folic acid, methionine and choline influence both DNA methylation and histone modification. Butyric acid is able to inhibit histone deacetylase and the more open structure resulting from acetylation has profound effects upon gene expression. Diallyl sulphide (DADS), the most prominent lipid-soluble organic sulphide compound in garlic, reduces turmourigenesis in rodents and may account for the anti-carcinogenic properties of garlic. Exposure of tumour cell lines to DADS inhibited histone deacetylase and resulted in increased acetylation of histones and the tumour cells exposed to DADS grew more slowly (Mathers, 2005).

The establishment of epigenetic changes in the genome may well be an important route for dietary ingredients to have a persistent influence upon the growth and development of an organism. However it is far from clear as to how the components of epigenetic marking of the genome interact to regulate gene expression and alter cell function.

Genomic stability

Diet is a key factor in determining the stability of the genome because it impacts on all relevant pathways, namely exposure to dietary carcinogens, activation or detoxification of carcinogens, DNA repair,

DNA synthesis and apoptosis (Fenech, 2002, 2003). A range of vitamins and minerals are required as cofactors for enzymes or as part of the structure of proteins involved in DNA metabolism. These include; vitamins C, E, B_2 $B_{6,}$ B_{12}, folate, niacin and the minerals Zn, Fe, Mg, and Mn. They play important roles in DNA synthesis and repair, in the prevention of oxidative damage to DNA, as well as in the maintenance of methylation of DNA (Fenech, 2003). An important point is that micronutrient deficiency can cause genome damage to the same extent as exposure to chemical carcinogens and ionising radiation.

The current Recommended Daily Allowance (RDA) for vitamins and minerals are based largely on the prevention of deficiency diseases. However in the modern world such diseases are relatively rare in both animals and humans whilst various non-infectious diseases and developmental diseases remain important. These are to some extent caused by damage to DNA. Therefore it would seem more logical to define optimal requirements of key nutrient and nutricines in terms of amounts to required to avoid damage to DNA. However at the present time the optimal nutrient and nutricine requirements for genomic stability have not been well established.

The concept of genome instability as a fundamental cause of disease offers a new approach for NbH. Genomic instability is preventable by adequate nutrition. Furthermore accurate diagnosis of genome instability using DNA damage biomarkers is technically feasible. Therefore it should be possible to optimise nutritional status and verify the efficacy of the strategy by diagnosis of a reduction in genome damage (see Chapter 8).

Genome to phenotype

The genome is clearly an important repository of basic information necessary for the growth and development of an animal. Therefore the stability of the genome and the degree of histone decoration and of methylation are all extremely important for health maintenance and disease avoidance. However, the genomic sequences only provide static information that does not describe the dynamic processes in living cells since all the nucleated cells in an organism contain exactly the same genetic information. They do not explain the complexity of living organisms nor provide information on the phenotype, or the physical form of the organism. In animal production it is the development of an appropriate phenotype which is desired. It is the expression of the genes in the cells of the body that generates the phenotype from the genotype. Consequently the ultimate result depends upon both the inherent nature of the genotype and on the expression of the genotype. This is an extremely complex process and is of necessity controlled at several different levels in eukaryotic cells.

The overall sequence of genome to phenotype starts with the transcription of DNA from an active gene and ends with the synthesis of proteins (Figure 2). Gene expression is mainly regulated at the initiation of the transcription of DNA into messenger RNA. This is the fundamental process whereby the genetic information encoded in DNA is first expressed. Expression of a gene is controlled by; numerous bioactive molecules, some species of RNA, hormones, and various transcription factors such as nuclear factor kappa B (NF-κB). Transcription factors select genes for activation or repression by recognizing the sequence of DNA bases in their promoter regions. Consequently, transcription factors are of great interest for their potential as therapeutic targets and as biological markers of disease states. Several external factors influence translation of mRNA into protein and then a multitude of post-translational modifications of proteins occur.

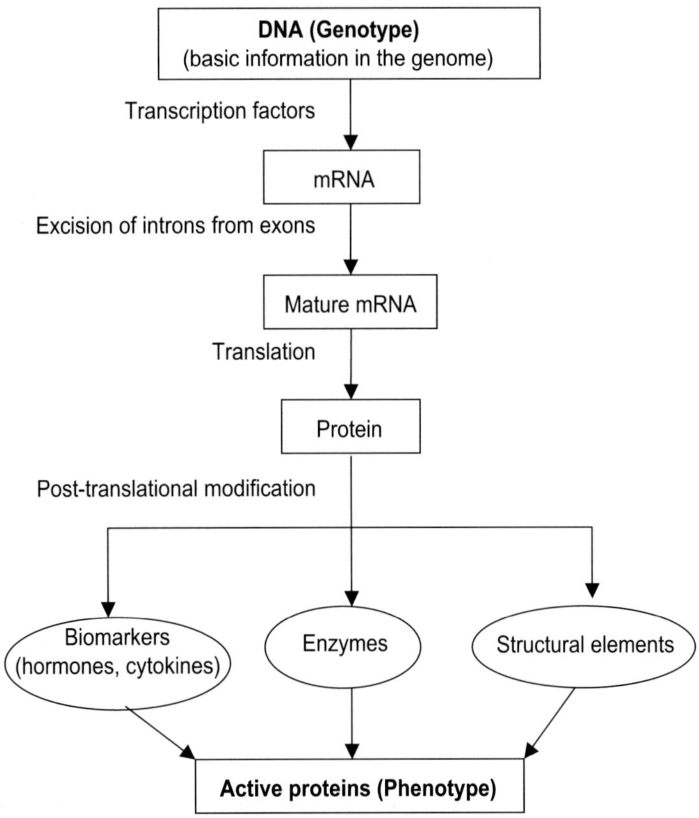

Figure 2. The progression from DNA (genotype) to active proteins (phenotype).

Nutrition and the regulation of mRNA translation

The control of mRNA translation also plays a key role in regulating gene expression under a wide range of circumstances in living cells.

The mRNA complement of a cell always provides a record of the proteins that are currently being synthesised. When cells need to increase rapidly the synthesis of particular proteins, the ability to up-regulate the translation of pre-existing mRNAs clearly allows the cell to start to make the corresponding protein without a requirement to activate transcription, process the resulting transcript and transport it to the cytoplasm. Situations requiring rapid increase in protein synthesis could be responses to nutrient availability and to stress.

Increases in the amounts or types of mRNA transcripts as a result of a nutritional or disease stress indicates up-regulation or induction of different genes as a response to the stress.

The synthesis of ferritin which is required for storage of iron is a good example of nutrition influencing mRNA translation. It is important to capture iron when available because it is essential for the production of haemoproteins such as haemoglobin and cytochromes, but also because iron ions are toxic and may catalyze oxidation reactions. Moreover bacterial virulence is greatly enhanced by freely available iron. Consequently natural resistance to infection requires free ionic iron to be virtually zero (Bullen *et al.*, 2005). Ferritin synthesis is rapidly enhanced in response to increased availability of iron, without a corresponding change in mRNA levels, indicating that iron enhances ferritin mRNA translation.

Role of environment

The inherent nature of the genotype is independent of the environment and is a fundamental characteristic of each animal species. It is the controlled expression in time and place of the many thousands of genes which make up the genome of the animal that directs the correct progression of growth and development, of health maintenance and of disease avoidance. However this expression of the genotype is inevitably influenced by the environment

A major source of environmental signals and stresses which influence gene expression is undoubtedly derived from feed ingredients, particularly the nutricines. Feed is not only an essential requirement for maintenance of life and health but it is also the largest source of chemicals that the cells of the body continuously encounter. At the basic biochemical, level feed consumption exposes cells on a regular basis to an enormous collection of heterogeneous molecules comprising, nutrients, nutricines, inert ingredients, micro-organisms and possible toxic materials.
There are also many variable environmental abiotic parameters such as temperature, pressure, oxygen, water availability, and variation in levels of ions, metals and numerous potentially toxic compounds.

To some extent variation in environmental conditions is easily accommodated but beyond certain limits stress is imposed, stimulating the animal to make metabolic adjustments that will counteract the negative effects of stress. Beyond these limits extreme environmental stress causes injury and even death.

The vigour and responsiveness of organisms to environmental stress results from a constant re-adjustment of physiology and metabolism throughout the life cycle of the organism within the framework of the genetic background. The genome-environmental interaction is therefore an essential focus for the elucidation of the nature of the phenotypic variation leading to a successful response to environmental stress. However the role that gene expression plays in response and adaptations to environmental stress is still not well established. Clearly stress-induced changes in protein types or protein concentrations must have arisen due to changes in the expression of appropriate genes.

Animals adapt to biotic and abiotic stresses by triggering a cascade or network of events that starts with stress perception and ends with the expression of a battery of target genes. The key components of the stress-response relationship are; stress stimulus, stress receptors, transducers, transcription regulators, target genes and stress responses. The ultimate response to various stresses will include morphological, biochemical and physiological changes (Pastori and Foyer, 2002).

Although the growth and development of an animal is due to a combination of genotype and to environmental effects, it is not always possible to differentiate the contribution of genotype from environmental factors. However amongst all the environmental factors that interact with the genotype, nutrition is perhaps the most important and plays a major role in animal growth.

This is very clearly demonstrated in the differential growth rates seen in broiler and layer chickens. The respective breeding and nutritional programmes for these two types of chickens result in broiler chickens on broiler feed being almost five times heavier than laying chickens fed a standard layer feed after six weeks of age (Zhao and Grossmann, 2002). Layer chickens increased weight by 35% when fed on broiler feed compared to those fed on layer feed. Conversely broiler chickens on layer feed had body weights reduced by 51% compared to those on broiler feed. Clearly the environmental effect, that is, feed type, plays a very important role in controlling body weight in addition to the effects of genotype.

This further suggests that nutritional regulation of gene expression is a major factor controlling animal growth. At the cellular level hypothalmic somatostatin (SS) mRNA was significantly higher in layer chickens on layer feed than in broiler chickens on broiler feed. Broiler feed down-regulated SS mRNA in layer chickens whereas layer feed up-regulated it in broiler chickens. Diets also had demonstrable effects upon pituitary growth hormone mRNA and liver growth hormone receptor gene expression.

The vigour and responsiveness of animals to environmental stress results from a constant re-adjustment of physiology and metabolism throughout the life cycle within the framework of the genetic background. The genome-environmental interaction is therefore an essential focus of future research for the elucidation of the nature of phenotypic variation in response to environmental cues. This is important since it is the characteristics of the phenotype which dictates the success or failure of animal production.

Nutrition and gene expression

Many bioactive food components have now been shown to have a direct effect upon gene expression. A clear example of a nutrient, glucose, on gene expression is illustrated in Figure 3 (Corthésy-Theulaz *et al.*, 2005). When carbohydrate from a feed is absorbed, it induces several metabolic events aimed at decreasing endogenous glucose production by the liver and increasing glucose storage and uptake in the form of glycogen and ultimately into lipids which are stored in adipose tissue. Conversely if glucose availability in the diet is reduced, glucose-utilizing pathways are inhibited and glucose–producing pathways are activated. These metabolic responses are facilitated by changes in gene expression levels. A high-carbohydrate diet induces the expression of several key glycolytic and lipogenic enzymes in the liver.

Many animal feeds typically contain large quantities of fats or oils that are heated or processed and these may develop high levels of peroxides which may have various undesirable metabolic effects and contribute to an oxidative stress. Thermally oxidised dietary fat was also able to activate gene expression in the liver (Sulzle *et al.*, 2004). Dietary oxidised fats led to an upregulation of genes encoding proteins involved in mitochondrial and peroxisomal ß-oxidation and hydroxylation of fatty acids. Furthermore this gene activation was not modified by supplementary vitamin E. Even moderate oxidative stress (*i.e.* non-cytotoxic) specifically down-regulates the expression of various genes (Morel and Barouki, 1999) and so oxidative stress may regulate gene expression as well as lead to the degradation of important molecules such as DNA and lipids.

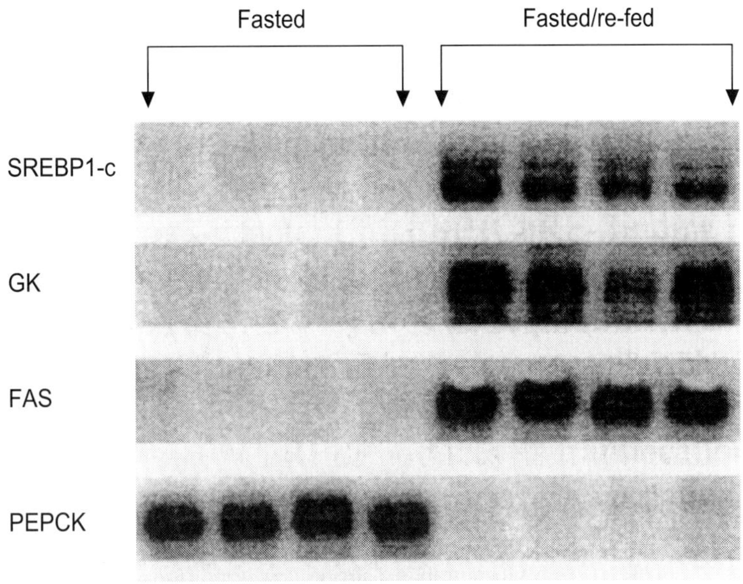

Figure 3.
Gene expression in liver of fasted rats and rats re-fed with a high-carbohydrate diet. The figure shows mRNA concentrations of the genes coding for the transcription factor, SREBP1-c, which mediates insulin action; glucokinase (GK), the first enzyme involved in glucose metabolism in hepatocytes; fatty acid synthase (FAS), which converts an excess of glucose into lipids; and phosphoenolpyuvate carboxykinase (PEPCK), which is a key enzyme of *de novo* glucose production (Corthésy-Theulaz *et al.*, 2005, permission granted by S. Karger AG)).

Phyto-oestrogens are multi-faceted compounds and the most extensively studied are the isoflavones which occur in soyabeans and a few other legumes. Most dietary sources contain a mixture of the isoflavones daidzein, genistein and glycitein (Figure 4). Isoflavones also occur in the form of glucosides, acetyl glucosides and malonyl glucosides.

There has been considerable interest over their activity in oestrogen-receptor mediated activities, particularly in relation to women's health (Cassidy, 2005). Traditionally, phyto-oestrogens have been considered as weakly oestrogenic and it is well established that the serum levels of isoflavones following consumption of a modest amount of soyabean-based foods can reach a concentration 100-1000 times that of oestradiol. Therefore, even if these compounds have a weak potency they have the potential to exert biological effects *in vivo*. It is not clear whether or not these phyto-oestrogens play a role in animal health.

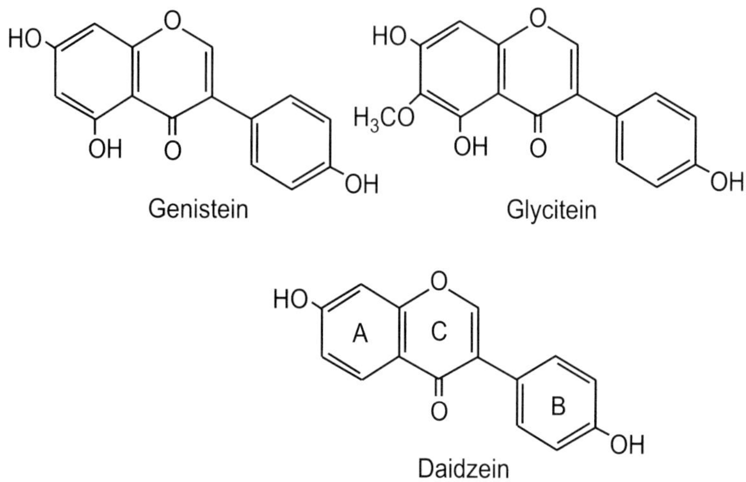

Figure 4.
Isoflavones.

Another example of a nutricine with many diverse molecular activities is curcumin (Lin and Lin-Shiau, 2001; Shapiro and Bruck, 2005). Curcumin is a strong colouring agent found in the spice tumeric which has long been used in various foods such as curries and mustards and is used in cosmetics and drugs. However the molecular mechanism of action of curcumin is quite complicated and diverse. It interacts with various targets at different levels from DNA in the genome to mRNA and influences enzyme activities. It is a potent scavenger of reactive oxygen species (ROS) and will help to protect lipids, haemoglobin and DNA from oxidative degradation. Curcumin seems to have multiple anti-tumour promoting effects. Curcumin increases the activities of the Phase 2 protective enzymes such as glutathione transferase, epoxide hydrolase, NADPH: quinone reductase and haem oxygenase whilst inhibiting procarcinogen activating Phase 1 enzymes, such as cytochrome P450.

The nutricines curcumin (Figure 5) and caffeic acid are potent inducers of haem oxygenase, which is a ubiquitous protein that protects cells against oxidative stress (Balogun *et al.*, 2003). It has an important role in degrading haem to CO, iron and biliverdin. Haem oxygenase activity is mediated through regulatory DNA sequences known as antioxidant-responsive elements. It appears that various nutricines can directly interact with the genome and so influence gene expression. This suggests a dual role for dietary antioxidants. They may protect tissues against oxidative stress by directly neutralizing reactive oxygen species in the classical antioxidant response and also by modulating gene expression.

Carotenoids are also capable of activating gene expression (Ruhl *et al.*, 2004). They interact with the pregnane X receptor which protects the organism against toxic substances.

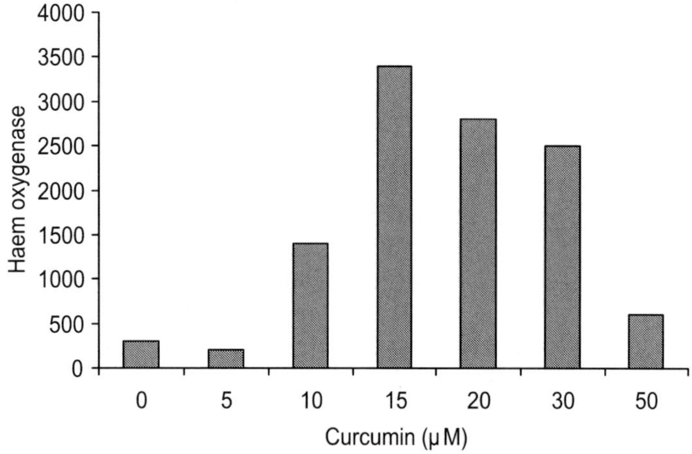

Figure 5. Effect of curcumin in stimulating haem oxyenase activity. (Reproduced with permission from Balogun *et al*, 2003).

The gene *hil*A in *Salmonella* is a regulator of pathogenicity and is directly involved in the invasion of intestinal epithelial cells. Medium-chain fatty acids are able to significantly decrease *hil*A expression which could have a positive benefit in reducing *Salmonella* invasion in poultry (Van Immerseel *et al.*, 2004).

There is considerable evidence now that inadequate foetal or neonatal nutrition influences gene expression (Langley-Evans, 2006). For example expression of the angiotensin II AT_2 receptor was modified by feeding a low-protein diet to gestating rats. DNA microarray studies have shown that the expression of 102 genes in the hypothalamus and 36 genes in the kidney are modified by intrauterine protein restriction. Although the association between nutrition and gene expression can be demonstrated it is not possible to ascertain whether these changes in gene expression are a cause of various disease syndromes or whether they are a consequence. Nevertheless it is clear that the nutritional status of an animal is associated with gene expression and with changes in the health/disease balance.

Soyabean protein is the major protein source for modern animal nutrition in both monogastric and poultry production. In pig production for example, it usually replaces the casein in sows milk at weaning and becomes the predominant protein source for the reminder of the life of the pig. It is quite intriguing to find that soyabean protein fed to rats with casein as a control showed distinct effects upon gene expression (Tachibana *et al.*, 2005). Gene expression in the liver of rats was investigated using DNA microarrays. In rats fed soyabean protein, 63 genes were up-regulated and 57 genes were down-regulated, compared to those fed casein. Most of these genes were involved in biochemical functions such as antioxidant activity, energy metabolism, lipid metabolism and transcriptional regulation. In lipid metabolism the down-regulated genes were related to fatty acid synthesis and the up-regulated genes were related to cholesterol synthesis and steroid catabolism. Soyabean protein is not only a useful source of dietary amino acids but possibly has some other beneficial effects in altering gene expression.

Transcription factors

Nuclear factor kappa B (NF-κB)

Another aspect of nutricines controlling metabolism is their effect on the activity of the transcription factor, NF-κB. This protein controls the transcription of mRNA for the pro-inflammatory cytokines such as tumour necrosis factor α (TNFα), interleukin-1ß (IL-1ß) and interleukin-6 (IL-6). It is normally kept inert in cells as an inactive complex with the inhibitory protein IκB. In response to external pro-inflammatory stimuli, a signalling cascade is activated, leading to phosphorylation and degradation of IκB and translocation of NF-κB to the nucleus where it initiates gene expression by binding to DNA.

Nuclear factor kappa B has a very wide spectrum of biochemical activities and is involved in activating or deactivating more than 175 genes in response to a wide range of substances and conditions. From its location in the cell cytoplasm NF-κB acts as a messenger, carrying outside signals to the nucleus and orchestrating the cell's response (Figure 6). It can stimulate the immune system which is clearly important in combating infectious diseases. Nuclear factor kappa B also plays an important role in inflammation which in turn is an important contributor to various non-infectious diseases such as heart problems, joint diseases and cancers.

Nuclear factor kappa B is highly active in inflammatory cells and abnormally active in some cancers (Marx, 2004). The evidence suggests that NF-κB promotes cancer by inhibiting apoptosis (programmed cell death) of cancer cells (Djavaheri-Mergny *et al.*, 2004). Curcumin inhibits the activation and binding of NF-κB to DNA and the subsequent transcription of pro-inflammatory molecules such as the cytokine TNF-α (Shapiro and Bruck, 2005). Gallates which are derivatives of the natural antioxidant gallic acid, exhibit anti-inflammatory properties *in vitro* by blocking activation of NF-κB (Murase *et al.*, 1999).

Possibly various nutricines such as antioxidants in red wine and green tea may have anti-cancer effects through an inhibition of NF-κB. Given the wide range of physiological effects controlled by NF-κB it is likely that an increasing number of dietary bioactive molecules or nutricines will be shown to play an important role in influencing NF-κB.

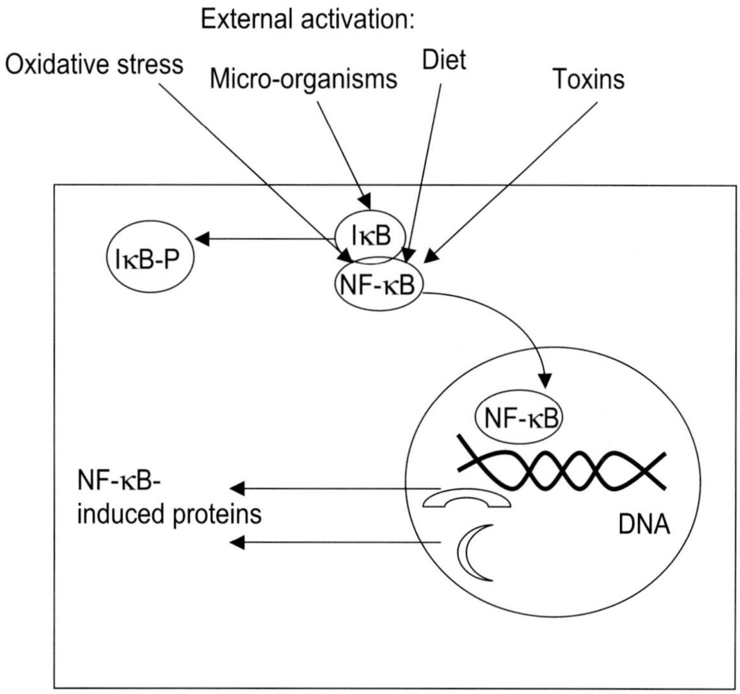

Figure 6. Many environmental effects activate NF-κB which leads to the synthesis of protective proteins.

Transcription factor –p53

The protein p53 is another transcription factor that is activated in response to a single-strand break in DNA, hypoxia, oxidative damage and nucleotide imbalance (Prives and Hall, 1999). It is thought to bind directly to sites of DNA damage and it may serve as a damage detector itself. Importantly p53 expression and activity are modulated at many levels within the cell. The main control areas are transcription, translation, post-translation including phosphorylation and acetylation, cellular localization and protein stability.

Following DNA injury cells express p53 induced proteins such as Bax and Bcl-2. The protein Bcl-2 is a survival protein and competes with Bax which is pro cell death. The Bcl-2:Bax ratio is therefore critical in determining sensitivity to cell death and eventual cell fate. Several factors can alter this ratio including calcium chelators such as EGTA (ethylene glycol tetraacetic acid) and BAPTA [bis-(o-aminophenoxy)ethane-*N, N, N′, N′*-tetra-acetic acid]. Fatal exposure of cells to EGTA or BAPTA resulted in a steady decrease in Bcl-2 mRNA levels whereas Bax mRNA increased in the 24 hours following exposure (Mizuno *et al.*, 1998).

When activated p53 can induce either growth arrest in a cell or initiate programmed cell death (apoptosis). Under conditions of little DNA damage, there is only a slight increase in the level of p53 expression and growth arrest is initiated to allow time for repair of the DNA. In the presence of large amounts of DNA damage p53 is highly expressed and cell death becomes inevitable.

Phytic acid which is a common constituent of animal feeds is also able to up-regulate the p53 gene (Saied and Shamsuddin, 1998). Consequently phytic acid has a novel anticancer action both *in vivo* and *in vitro*. It inhibits cell growth, decreases cell proliferation and also causes differentiation of various cancer cell lines.

Generally in animal nutrition phytic acid is considered as an unavailable source of phosphorus and phytase enzymes are routinely added to animal feeds in order to hydrolyze the phytic acid into available phosphorus. However it is curious to see that phytic acid might be a useful nutricine in activating the production of the transcription factor p53. Furthermore phytic acid also seems to have beneficial effects on colon morphology (Jenab and Thompson, 2000).

Nutritional genomics (nutrigenomics)

With the elucidation of the sequence of various genomes and the recent developments in proteomic technologies it is now possible to study gene regulation and gene function in relation to nutrition (Mathers, 2004). Nutritional genomics or nutrigenomics, therefore attempts to study the influences of nutrition upon the expression of the genome. This must consider the interaction between the changing nutritional environment of cells and the static genome. Nutritional genomics is concerned with the systematic assessment of how nutricines modify the overall gene expression patterns in cells and tissues of interest. Nutricines can activate or inactivate gene products and in effect play a role as metabolic switches.

Studies in nutritional genomics should help to elucidate of the differences among nutricines in relation to the gene expression response. The practical implication of nutrigenomics is an attempt to provide a genetic and molecular understanding of how common dietary chemicals, particularly nutricines, affect the balance between health and disease by altering the expression of and possibly the structure of an individual's genetic make-up (Kaput, 2004). The challenge of nutritional genomics is therefore to understand how dietary components influence gene expression and how they can offset the negative effect of the numerous environmental insults to which a living organism is continuously exposed.

Nutricine genomics offers several strategies to probe the interactions between diet and health. For example by focusing on the disease state and tracking back through the mechanism of development it should be possible to identify the earliest genes involved in the disease process. These genes might then be used as targets to identify nutricines that are capable of modulating their expression, thus eliminating the disease formation process (Elliot and Ong, 2002).

An alternative approach would be to start with the healthy state and examine the effects of nutricines on global patterns of gene expression. Specific effects of diet on patterns of gene expression would provide the focus to understand disease development processes. This in turn would lead to an improvement in the understanding of the impact of nutrition on health, and could guide nutritional programmes.

Conclusions

The genome, which is the repository of all the genetic information in a cell or tissue can be modified through changes to the histone proteins or by DNA methylation. These modifications are epigenetic changes which are essential for normal development and can be influenced by dietary components. Nutrition also affects genomic stability which is a fundamental cause of disease. Many dietary compounds influence the sequence from genotype to phenotype. They can influence gene expression and the synthesis of mRNA. The expression of the phenotype is an interaction between genotype and environment. Feed ingredients may directly affect gene expression or they may act through the activation of transcription factor systems that regulate specific sets of genes in different tissues and under different environmental conditions. The relationship between nutrition and expression of the genotype, or nutrigenomics, has important practical implications. It is an attempt to provide a genetic and molecular understanding for how common dietary chemicals, particularly nutricines, affect the balance between health and disease. This in turn would lead to an improvement in the understanding of the impact of nutrition on health, and could guide nutritional programmes.

References

Avramova, Z. V. (2002). Heterochromatin in animals and plants. Similarities and differences. *Plant Physiology*, 129: 40-49.

Balogun, E., Hoque, M., Gong, H., Killeen, E., Green, C. J., Foresti, R., Alam, J. and Motterlini, R. (2003). Curcumin activates the haem oxygenase-1 gene via regulation of Nrf2 and the antioxidant –responsive element. *Biochemical Journal*, 371: 887-895.

Boffa, L. C., Lupton, J. R., Mariani, M. R., Ceppi, M., Newmark, H. L., Scalmati, A. and Lipkin, M. (1992). Modulation of colonic epithelial cell proliferation, histone acetylation, and luminal short chain fatty acids by variation of dietary fibre (wheat bran) in rats.

Cancer Research, **52**: 5906-5912.

Bullen, J. J., Rogers, H. J., Spalding, P. B. and Ward, C. G. (2005). Iron and infection: the heart of the matter. *FEMS Immunology and Medical Microbiology*, **43**: 325-330.

Cassidy, A. (2005). Dietary phyto-oestrogens: molecular mechanisms, bioavailability and importance to menopausal health. *Nutrition Research Reviews*, **18**: 183-201.

Corthésy-Theulaz, I., den Dunnen, J. T., Ferré, P., Geurts, J. M. W., Müller, M., van Belzen, N. and van Ommen, B. (2005). Nutrigenomics: The impact of biomics technology on nutrition research. *Annals of Nutrition and Metabolism*, **49**: 355-365.

Djavaheri-Mergny, M., Javelaud, D., Wietzerbin, J. and Besançon, F. (2004). NF-kB activation prevents apotoptic oxidative stress via an increase of both thioredoxin and MnSOD levels in TNFa-treated Ewing sarcoma cells. *FEBS Letters*, **578**: 111-115.

Eden, A., Gaudet, F., Waghmare, A. and Jaenisch, R. (2003). Chromosomal instability and tumors promoted by DNA hypomethylation. *Science*, **300**: 455.

Elliot, R. and Ong, T. J. (2002). Nutritional genomics. *British Medical Journal*, **324**: 1438-1442.

Fang, M. Z., Wang, Y., Ai, N., Hou, Z., Sun, Y., Hong, L., Welsh W. and Yang, C. S. (2003). Tea polyphenol (-)epigallocatechin inhibits DNA methyltransferase and reactivates methylation-silenced genes in cancer cell lines. *Cancer Research*, **63**: 7563-7570.

Fang, M. Z., Chen, D., Sun, Y., Jin, Z., Christman, J. K., and Yang, C. S. (2005). Reversal of hypermethylation and reactivation of $p16^{INK4a}$, *RARß*, and MGMT genes by genistein and other isoflavones from soy. *Clinical Cancer Research*, **11**: 7033-7041.

Fenech, M. (2002). Micronutrients and genomic stability: a new paradigm for recommended daily allowances (RDAs). *Food and Chemical Toxicology*, **40**: 1113-1117.

Fenech, M. (2003). Nutritional treatment of genome instability: a paradigm shift in disease prevention and in the setting of recommended dietary allowances. *Nutrition Research Reviews*, **16**: 109-122.

Gaudet, F., Hodgson, J. G., Eden, A., Jackson-Grusby, L., Dausman, J., Gray, J. W., Leonhardt, H. and Jaenisch, R. (2003). Induction of tumours in mice by genomic hypomethylation. *Science*, **300**: 489-492.

Jenab, M. and Thompson, L. U. (2000). Phytic acid in wheat bran affects colon morphology, cell differentiation and apoptosis. *Carcinogenesis*, **21**: 1547-1552.

Kaput, J. (2004). Diet-disease gene interactions. *Nutrition*, **20**: 26-31.

Langley-Evans, S. C. (2006). Developmental programming of health and disease. *Proceedings of the Nutrition Society*, **65**: 97-105.

Lee, H. S. and Chen, Z. J. (2001). Protein-coding genes are

epigenetically regulated in Arabidopsis polyploids. *Proceedings of the National Academy of Science (USA)*, **98**: 6753-6758.

Lin, J-K. and Lin-Shiau, S-Y. (2001). Mechanisms of cancer chemoprevention by curcumin. *Proceedings of the National Science Council, ROC (B)*, **25**: 59-66.

Marx, J. (2004). Inflammation and cancer: the link grows stronger. *Science*, **306**: 966-968.

Mathers , J. C. (2004). What can we expect to learn from genomics? *Proceedings of the Nutrition Society* **63**:1-4.

Mathers, J. C. (2005). Nutrition and epigenetics – how the genome learns from experience. *British Nutrition Foundation Nutrition Bulletin*, **30**: 6-12.

McCabe, D. C. and Caudill, M. A. (2005). DNA methylation, genomic silencing, and links to nutrition and cancer. *Nutrition Reviews*, **63**: 183-195.

Mizuno, N., Yoshitomi, H., Ishida, H., Kuromi, H., Kawaki, J., Seino, Y. and Seino, S. (1998). Altered bcl-2 and bax expression and intracellular calcium signalling in apoptosis of pancreatic cells and the impairment of glucose-induced insulin secretion. *Endocrinology*, **139**: 1429-1439.

Morel, Y. and Barouki, R. (1999). Repression of gene expression by oxidative stress. *Biochemical Journal*, **342**: 481-496.

Murase, T., Kume, N., Hase, T., Shibuya, Y., Nishizawa, Y., Tokimutsu, I. and Kita, T. (1999). Gallates inhibit cytokine-induced nuclear translocation of NF-κB and expression of leukocyte adhesion molecules in vascular endothelial cells. *Arteriosclerosis, Thrombosis and Vascular Biology*, **19**: 1412-1420.

Pastori, G. A. and Foyer, C. H. (2002). Common components, networks and pathways of cross-tolerance to stress. The central role of "redox" and abscisic acid-mediated controls. *Plant Physiology*, **129**: 460-468.

Pennisi, E. (2005). Why do humans have so few genes? *Science*, **309**: 80.

Prives, C. and Hall, P. A. (1999). The p53 pathway. *Journal of Pathology*, **187**: 112-126

Ruhl, R., Sczech, R., Landes, N., Pfluger, K., Kluth, D. and Schweigert, F. J. (2004). Carotenoids and their metabolites are naturally occurring activators of gene expression via the pregnane X receptor. *European Journal of Nutrition*, **43**: 336-343.

Saied, I. T. and Shamsuddin, A. M. (1998). Up-regulation of the tumor suppressor gene p53 and WAFI gene expression by IP6 in HT-29 human colon carcinoma cell line. *Anticancer Research*, **18**: 1479-1484.

Shapiro, H. and Bruck, R. (2005). Therapeutic potential of curcumin in non-alcoholic steatohepatitis. *Nutrition Research Reviews*, **18**: 212-221.

Strahl, B. D. and Allis, C. D. (2000). The language of covalent histone modifications. *Nature*, **403**: 41-45.

Sulzle, A., Hirche, F. and Eder, K. (2004). Thermally oxidised dietary fat upregulates the expression of target genes of PPAR-alpha in rat liver. *Journal of Nutrition*, **143**: 1375-1383.

Tachibana, N., Matsumoto, I., Fukui, K., Arai, S., Kato, H., Abe, K. and Takamatsu, K. (2005). Intake of soy protein isolate alters hepatic gene expression in rats. *Journal of Agricultural and Food Chemistry*, **53**: 4253-4257.

Van Immerseel, F., De Buck, J., Boyen, F., Bohez, L., Pasmans, F., Volf, J., Sevcik, M., Rychlik, I., Hasebrouck, F. and Ducatelle, R. (2004); Medium-chain fatty acids decrease colonization and invasion through *hilA* suppression shortly after infection of chickens with *Salmonella enterica* serovar enteritidis. *Applied and Environmental Microbiology*, **70**: 3582-3587.

Zhao, R. and Grossmann, R. (2002). Regulation of growth in poultry: impact of nutrition. 11th European Poultry Conference, *Archiv für Geflügelkunder*, **66**: 38.

3 Feed-Pathogen Interactions

An important series of disease syndromes arise when pathogenic micro-organisms invade the gastrointestinal tract and ultimately the cells of the body of the animal. It is now established that an essential first step for the pathogenesis of certain bacteria which may cause enteric diseases is adhesion to the cells of the wall of the gastrointestinal tract. The second stage in development of enteric disease is then the proliferation of the pathogen in the gastrointestinal tract. Therefore the basic objectives in the development of NbH must be to identify and to exploit various feed raw materials and other bioactive feed ingredients, nutricines (Adams, 1999; Adams, 2002), to inhibit pathogen adhesion, to inhibit pathogen growth and to ensure that the diet does not increase the virulence of pathogens.

Pathogen adhesion

It is widely accepted that adhesion of enteric, oral and respiratory bacteria is required for colonization and subsequent development of disease. Moreover, bacteria assume a significantly greater resistance to killing by immune factors, bacteriolytic enzymes and antibiotics when they have adhered to tissue surfaces. Bacteria which have successfully adhered to a tissue surface are better able to acquire nutrients which further enhances their ability to survive and provoke an infectious disease. Bacterial adhesion then is a key stage in pathogenesis. Therefore prevention of bacterial adhesion soon after exposure of the host to the pathogen should lead to disease avoidance (Ofek *et al.*, 2003).

Pathogen adhesion usually occurs through the recognition of host cell receptors by the bacteria. These host cell receptors are often cell-surface oligosaccharides.

Such oligosaccharides can also be conjugated to proteins from dairy food such as caseinoglycomacropeptide obtained from milk. If these molecules are present in the gastrointestinal tract they may act as decoys for the pathogenic bacteria. This offers an interesting possibility of the control of infection by means of incorporating anti-adhesive molecules into the diet in order to reduce the adhesion of common gastrointestinal pathogens.

Caseinoglycomacropeptide exerted some anti-adhesive properties in a model system using human cells in culture (Rhoades *et al.*, 2006) (Table1). The caeinoglycmacropeptide was able to reduce the adhesion of non-toxigenic strains of *Escherichia coli* to less than 50% of the control and reduced adhesion of enteropathogenic strains to between 80 and 10% of the control. However the caseinoglycomacropeptide also reduced the adhesion of some *Lactobacilli* species so this would probably reduce its effectiveness as a dietary treatment. In general the anti-adhesive effects of a feed component would need to be selective for pathogens over the desirable microflora in the gastrointestinal tract.

Table 1. The effect of caseinglycomacropeptide on the adhesion of bacteria to human cells in culture.

Micro-organisms tested	*Adhesion relative to control (%)*
Escherichia coli 12900 (non toxigenic)	51
E. coli 13127 (non toxigenic)	46
E. coli 13128 (non toxigenic)	31
E. coli O111:H27 (enteropathogenic)	87
E. coli O110: H4 (enteropathogenic)	37
E. coli O128 H12 (enteropathogenic	4
Lactobacillus pentosus	44
L. acidophilus	81
L. casei	42

Cranberry juice has also been shown to contain at least two anti-adhesive agents (Ofek *et al.*, 2003). One is probably a large molecular weight tannin and the other is a protoanthocyanidin. The tannin inhibited the adhesion to animal cells of uropathogenic *E.coli* but did not act on the adhesion of *E. coli* causing diarrhea. This may well explain the benefits of cranberry juice in controlling urinary infections.

Non-digestible oligosaccharides based on the sugar mannose may also offer protection by acting as ligands for pathogenic bacteria and preventing their adhesion to or invasion of the wall of the gastrointestinal tract. Results with turkeys indicated that mannanoligosaccharides improved performance comparable to that seen with antibiotic growth promoters (Parks *et al.*, 2001). This improvement in performance may be due to a reduction in the pathogen load encountered by the birds under farm conditions although this was not directly demonstrated and would be difficult to do.

The development of an anti-adhesion therapy based on feed ingredients is an attractive means for health maintenance and disease avoidance in animals. A practical advantage in obtaining anti-adhesion molecules from feed ingredients is that toxicity is not likely to be much of an issue. However there are still major difficulties in obtaining anti-adhesion compounds which would have a broad specificity and be economical for use in animal feeds.

Inhibit pathogen growth

Feed raw materials

There is scattered evidence that various feed raw materials have useful characteristics in terms of inhibiting growth of pathogens in the gastrointestinal tract of animals.

Pigs

In pig production weaning at three to four weeks of age is widely recognised as a stress for piglets, characterised by a reduction in feed intake, growth rate and feed conversion efficiency. This is frequently manifested as disturbances of the gastrointestinal microflora and detrimental changes in gut morphology which generally results in reduced growth rates. Antibiotics have been widely used in the recent past in young pig diets as a means of alleviating some of these digestive disorders. However all antibiotic growth promoters used in feed were banned in the EU in January 2006 so there is now considerable increased interest in NbH to compensate for the loss of the antibiotics.

Diets for early-weaned piglets usually contain high levels of protein which may encourage proliferation of pathogenic bacteria in the gastrointestinal tract. This may well contribute to increased post-weaning diarrhoea problems in weaned piglets. One possible solution to this problem is to reduce the amount of protein in piglet feeds and to supplement with various amino acids. This could reduce the amount of substrate available for bacterial growth in the gastrointestinal tract which would subsequently benefit piglet health.

Diets with low nutrient content, only 8.9% crude protein, compared to a standard of 18%, and with high fibre remarkably reduced the severity of *E.coli* enterotoxaemia in weaned pigs (Bertschinger *et al.,* 1979). There was no mortality due to enterotoxaemia compared to a rate of 26% in the control animals. The addition of herring meal, which is a good source of digestible protein, neutralized the protective effect of the diet suggesting that low protein in the diets was the important factor. High protein diets are frequently not thoroughly utilized by the weaned pig during the digestion process. This leaves excess protein in the gastrointestinal tract which can be utilized by bacteria such as *E. coli.*

In another study lowering the protein content of piglet diets from 23% to 19% reduced final body weight, overall average daily gain and feed conversion ratio (Nyachoti *et al.*, 2006) which are clearly undesirable effects from the general production point of view. However there were also potential ancillary health benefits in that the pH and ammonia level in the digesta was reduced with low protein diets (Table 2). The high protein feed with 23% CP gave the highest digesta pH and this is likely to provide a more favourable environment for the growth of enteric pathogens such as *Escherichia coli* than a lower pH as found with reduced protein diets. There was a very significant reduction in ammonia in the digesta from reduced protein diets. This may reduce the metabolic stress on the animals associated with ammonia detoxification in the liver.

Table 2. The effect of reduced dietary protein on the pH and ammonia level in the digesta of piglets in various regions of the gastrointestinal tract.

Digesta parameter	*Dietary crude protein (%)*	*Duodenum*	*Jejunum*	*Ileum*
pH	23	5.88	6.32	6.74
	21	5.65	6.01	6.02
	19	5.96	6.06	6.09
Ammonia in digesta (mg/L)	23	17.68	35.28	71.96
	21	13.78	33.57	49.26
	19	10.70	27.08	42.45

Feeding diets with a reduced nitrogen content does not necessarily reduce the performance of growing pigs if the amino acid balance is well managed (Tuitoek *et al.*, 1997). Reducing dietary crude protein content in feed from 16.6 %t o 13.0% for pigs from 20-55kg had no significant effect upon average daily gain, feed conversion ration or protein deposition. There may well be health benefits from modest reductions in the protein contents of piglet and pig diets which will not impact adversely upon economic performance.

Post weaning collibacillosis (PWC) is a multifactorial disease of piglets and its expression is influenced by nutrition (Pluske *et al.*, 2002). Feeding a diet based on cooked white rice and animal protein sources was very protective against the development of PWC (McDonald *et al.*, 1999). A similar protective effect of cooked rice and animal protein was also seen in pigs experimentally infected with the intestinal spirochete, *Brachyspira hyodysenteriae*, the agent of swine dysentery, (Pluske *et al.*, 1996). These results however could not be repeated in European studies (Lindecrona *et al.*, 2003). In this work a diet based on cooked rice with a low content of non-starch polysaccharides and resistant starch did not prevent the development of swine dysentry upon experimental challenge with *B. hyodysenteriae*. The best results were obtained from feeding a fermented liquid feed. However more recent work, in this case with *E. coli* in piglets, again confirmed the beneficial effect of a cooked rice and protein diet (Montagne *et al.*, 2004). In this study animal protein could also be replaced by plant protein and the protective effect of the diet did not diminish. Furthermore addition of carboxymethylcellulose to cooked white rice increased digesta viscosity and enhanced the post weaning collibacillosis indicating that diet plays a role in the incidence of this enteric disorder.

The protective effects of these diets against bacterial infection has been attributed in part to the high digestibility of the carbohydrate in the boiled rice and of the animal protein (McDonald *et al.,* 1999, Pluske *et al.,* 1996). Nutrients from well-digested feed ingredients would be rapidly absorbed out of the gastrointestinal tract. This would limit the amount of fermentable substrate in the lower small intestine and reduce that entering the large intestine where the majority of the gastrointestinal microflora reside. This explanation is further supported by the results with carboxymethyl cellulose. Increased viscosity of the digesta reduces the efficiency of digestion and absorption of nutrients and thus leaves more nutrients available for pathogenic bacteria.

The use of cooked rice as a replacement for cooked maize in piglet diets increased feed intake, nutrient digestibility and piglet performance (Mateos *et al.*, 2006). However it did not reduce the proportion of animals needing treatment for diarrhoea for at least two consecutive days but the proportion of days with diarrhoea with respect to the total number of days on trial was reduced from 9.0 with maize to 3.2 with cooked rice. The higher feed intake of 659 g/day with cooked rice compared to 623 g/day with cooked maize might also give an advantage to the piglets in their early growth phase where feed intake is an important health and performance indicator. It seems that where possible cooked rice would be a valuable ingredient in diets for piglets.

llieitis, or porcine proliferative enteropathy, is an important enteric disease of pigs that decreases feed intake and growth rates and increases mortality. The disease is caused by the bacterium *Lawsonia intracellularis* that infects the enterocytes in the gastrointestinal tract. The disease is difficult to treat and is a continuous problem in modern pig production.

There has been a considerable amount of work done on using distillers dried grains in pig diets at 10-20% in an attempt to reduce the severity of *ilieitis* (Whitney *et al.*, 2006). However in three disease challenge studies only one gave a positive response to the inclusion of dried distillers grains in the feed. The ability of the pig to resist a disease challenge through nutritional manipulation is probably related to the severity of the challenge and it seems that distillers dried grains gave at best only minimal benefits against *ilieitis* when severely challenged.

Catlle

Switching cattle feed from grain to hay was also associated with a reduction in *E.coli* 0157:H7 (Callaway, *et al.,* 2003). This micro-organism is not a pathogen for cattle but causes haemorrhagic colitis in humans which can be fatal. An abrupt switch in cattle feeding from grain to hay is in many cases not practical even though there are clear human health benefits in terms of food safety. Nevertheless it does suggest future research strategies and indicates that nutritional solutions to such problems are possible.

Poultry

A major food safety problem today is *Campylobacter jejuni* which is carried asymptomatically in the gastrointestinal tract of many food animals, particularly broiler chickens (Mead, 2002; Park, 2002). There is rapid horizontal transmission of *Campylobacter* in broiler flocks that leads to heavy contamination of broiler carcasses after processing (Shanker *et al.*, 1990). Although *Campylobacter* is common in broilers the origin of infection is still not clear. When feed was deliberately contaminated by *Campylobacter* and stored at room temperature, no culturable cells were recovered after 48 hours (Mills and Phillips, 2003) which suggests that survival of the organism in feeds is unlikely. *Campylobacter* is sensitive to desiccation, high oxygen tension, high and low temperatures. Consequently modern feed manufacturing, transport and storage systems are unlikely to be congenial for *Campylobacter*. If it is not feed-borne, then general feed hygiene procedures may not solve the problem. Nevertheless the organism occurs in the gastrointestinal tract and probably feed-based treatments will be needed to control *Campylobacter* and improve food safety.

Feed raw materials have some effect upon *Campylobacter* (Udayamputhoor *et al.*, 2003). Birds consuming feed made from plant-based protein sources; soyabean meal, canola meal and maize gluten meal, had less *Campylobacter* than birds consuming feed based on animal protein sources; meat meal, poultry by-product meal, fishmeal and feather meal (Table 3).

Table 3. *Campylobacter* shedding and intestinal contamination in broilers on feeds from animal- or plant-based protein sources.

Protein source	*Shedding (%)*	*Campylobacter counts*	
		Caecum	*Jejuni*
Animal	85.7	6.3	3.4
Plant	66.6	4.9	2.8

The lower level of colonization in the birds fed plant protein may be explained in terms of a combined influence of various substrates in the diet. Plant protein-based feeds contain various non-starch polysaccharides which may be fermented in the caeca into organic acids which would be detrimental to *Campylobacter*. Iron is an essential micronutrient for the growth of *Campylobacter* and plant-protein based feeds are likely to be poorer in available iron than animal-protein based feeds.

Other plant materials, not commonly used in modern animal nutrition, such as leek, garlic and onion have anti-*Campylobacter* effects (Lee *et al.*, 2004). These data suggest that feed raw materials of plant origin might be useful in control of *Campylobacter*.

Coccidiosis, an important disease of poultry, is influenced by feed ingredients (Persia *et al.*, 2006). Both acute and chronic coccidiosis infection reduced growth performance, ME and amino acid digestibility in chicks fed a conventional maize-soyabean meal. When the soyabean meal was partially replaced by 15% of fishmeal the response to coccidiosis infection was much reduced (Table 4). The fish oil fraction of the fishmeal may have given beneficial effects in terms of reducing the inflammatory response to coccidiosis infection. The omega-3 fatty acids in fish oils are recognised as having anti-inflammatory properties.

Table 4. Growth performance of chicks inoculated with sporulated *Eimeria acervulina* oocysts and given feeds based on maize/soyabean meal or on maize/soyabean meal/fishmeal.

Feed	*Infection with E. acervulina*	*Weight gain (g)*	*Feed intake (g)*	*FCR*
Maize/soya	Control (sham)	357	508	1.42
	Acute	310	486	1.56
	Chronic	322	469	1.46
Maize/soya/fish	Control (sham)	365	499	1.37
	Acute	349	490	1.40
	Chronic	361	492	1.36

Nutricines

Animal feeds contain many bioactive components, nutricines, in additional to the classical nutrients. Nutricines such as antioxidants, carotenoids and organic acids, are increasingly being used in a NbH strategy. The effects of antioxidants and carotenoids is further discussed in Chapters 6 and 7.

Organic acids

There are many different organic acids commercially available either as the free acids or in the form of various ammonium, calcium, potassium or sodium salts (Table 5). This makes their practical application somewhat confusing. Generally the acids are all small molecules with molecular weights less than 200.

Many organic acids such as; acetic, butryric, citric, fumaric and lactic and propionic are natural components of feeds, or are produced in the gastrointestinal tract through fermentation of non-digestible carbohydrates. These organic acids are basically non-toxic to cells of animals or humans even at high dose rates, but they are quite toxic to cells of micro-organisms at relatively low dose rates. In the gastrointestinal tract they may also

Table 5. Various acids and acid salts used in feeds.

Acetic	Fumaric
Benzoic	Lactic
Potassium benzoate	Calcium lactate
Sodium benzoate	Phosphoric
Sodium butyrate	Propionic
Citric	Ammonium propionate
Sodium citrate	Calcium propionate
Formic	Sorbic
Calcium formate	Potassium sorbate
Potassium formate	Tartaric

encourage the growth of non-pathogenic bacteria by acting as a substrate or carbon source and they also inhibit the growth of pathogenic bacteria. Consequently organic acids have now become a very important group of nutricines following the prohibition of antibiotic growth promoters and increasing concerns on feed hygiene in the EU. They may play a valuable role in NbH. They have been widely used piglet and pig feeds with good effect in terms of reducing gastrointestinal problems (Partanen & Mroz, 1999).

Butyric acid is quite interesting as it has bactericidal activity and also plays a role in development of the intestinal epithelium. It is quite important for the normal development of epithelial cells (Pryde *et al.*, 2002) and is the major energy source for the enterocytes. Free butyric acid is difficult to use in feed manufacture because of its' unpleasant odour. Furthermore the free acid is likely to be rapidly metabolized in the upper digestive tract and is unlikely to reach the large intestine. To overcome these problems butyric acid was studied in the form of a mixture of mono-, di-, and triglycerides (Leeson *et al.*, 2005). An incorporation of 0.2% butyric acid into broiler feeds helped to maintain the performance and carcass quality of broilers challenged with coccidiosis.

Turkey poult enteritis and mortality syndrome (PEMS) is a major economic threat to turkey production in the USA. The syndrome is caused by agents such as bacteria and viruses that irritate and injure the intestines of young turkeys. An immune dysfunction is also frequently associated with PEMS which increases susceptibility to secondary bacterial infections that ultimately kill the poult. Treatment of feed for turkey poults with a propionic acid-based mixture at 1.25% did not prevent the disease occurring in the PEMS-challenged poults. However it did reduce the cumulative mortality by 50% (Fig. 1) (Roy *et al.*, 2002), and produced a delay in the onset of the initial mortality spike. The addition of organic acids at 1.25% to the feed would decrease the microbial contamination in the feed and also decrease the bacterial load in the intestine and caeca. Therefore, it is likely that the overall pathogenic challenge to the birds was decreased and this may have resulted in the reduced mortality shown in Fig. 1.

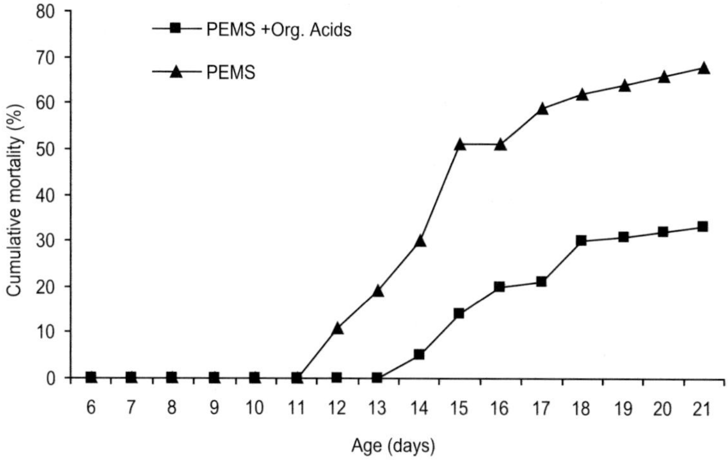

Figure 1. Percentage cumulative mortality for poults challenged with PEMS on day 6.

Contamination of eggs, poultry meat and pig meat by *Salmonella* is a serious public health issue and needs to be avoided and controlled in the animal production process. Animal nutrition plays an important role in *Salmonella* control due to its effects on the microflora in the gastrointestinal tract (Coma, 2003). Pigs fed pelleted and dry feeds are more susceptible to *Salmonella* contamination than pigs fed wet mash feed. The advantage of wet feeding is thought to be due to the formation of organic acids by fermentation in the wet feed. However feed particle size can also influence *Salmonella* contamination, with coarse mash feed being most protective against *Salmonella*. This again seems to stimulate production of lactic, acetic, propionic and butyric acids in the gastrointestinal tract. This is turn is associated with larger population of *Lactobacilli* and lower coliform numbers (Coma, 2003).

Medium chain fatty acids (MCFA) have been considered as a potential alternative for antibiotic growth promoters in pig nutrition (Dierick *et al.*, 2002). Further studies with MCFA showed that they had some antimicrobial activity against *Salmonella* and the antibacterial activity appeared to be higher than that of the short chain fatty acids such as formic, acetic, propionic and butyric (Van Immerseel *et al.*, 2004a).

An important pathogen for pigs is *Lawsonia intracellularis* which causes porcine proliferative enteropathy. Pigs given feed supplemented with 2.4% lactic acid had significantly reduced pathogenic lesions in the intestines four weeks post infection (Boesen *et al.*, 2004), although lactic acid was not able to reduce infection with *Brachyspira hyodysenteriae* (Lindecrona *et al.*, 2003).

Organic acids, routinely used in a wide variety of poultry and pig feeds to alleviate various enteric problems, are frequently described as "acidifiers" but this is in reality a misnomer. Organic acids in feed only slightly reduce the pH of the feed and they do not dramatically shift the pH of the gastrointestinal tract which is a highly buffered system. This is illustrated in Table 6, where feeds with either 1.5% fumaric or 1.5% citric acid were given to piglets (Risley *et al.*, 1991). The organic acids did not reduce the pH in either the gastric digesta or in the digesta of the other intestinal sections. These observations were confirmed by Canibe *et al.*, (2005) who found that the pH of the digesta from pigs given feed with 1.8% formic acid was only slightly reduced in the stomach but not in the rest of the gastrointestinal tract. Clearly the beneficial effect of organic acids in terms of animal growth and performance is not due to an acidification *per se* of the digesta in the gastrointestinal tract. Nevertheless these nutricines still exert an influence upon pathogenic bacteria resident in the gastrointestinal tract.

Table 6. Gastrointestinal pH in eight-week old piglets given either 1.5% fumaric or 1.5% citric acids in feed.

Section of gastrointestinal tract	*Treatment*		
	Control	*Fumaric acid*	*Citric acid*
Stomach	4.73	4.30	4.83
Jejunum	7.06	7.01	7.00
Caecum	5.96	6.04	6.05
Lower colon	6.51	6.53	6.47

The precise mode of action of these acids as antimicrobials is still not established (Cherrington *et al.*, 1990). At low external pH values the undissociated organic acid molecule is lipophilic and readily enters the microbial cell and then dissociates into a proton and anion. Both the protons and the anions have inhibitory effects upon the microbial cell which include; provoking a collapse of the cell membrane potential (Eklund, 1985) and reduction in the rates of RNA, DNA, protein, lipid and cell wall synthesis (Cherrington *et al.*, 1990). However in the gastrointestinal tract distal to the stomach the pH of the digesta (Table 6), is above the general pKa of the organic acids and so perhaps the effect is due more to the effects of the anions.

Chlorate

Another route to reduce *E. coli* O157:H7 populations in live animals is by feeding sodium chlorate (Edrington, *et al.*, 2003). The enzyme nitrate reductase, which is present in *E. coli*, will use chlorate as an anologue of nitrate. The chlorate will be reduced to the toxic metabolite chlorite which kills the bacterial cells. A chlorate-based product has been successfully tested against *Salmonella* contamination in broilers

(Byrd *et al.*, 2003). Sodium chlorate has low toxicity for animals but such a nutritional strategy would probably face serious regulatory obstacles.

Enzymes

Rapid digestion and absorption of nutrients is certainly an important aspect of NbH as this reduces the amount of substrate remaining in the gastrointestinal tract which could be used by pathogenic micro-organisms. Considerable progress has already been made in this area with enzymes (Bedford, 2000) and lysophospholipids (Schwarzer & Adams, 1996; Xing *et al.*, 2004). Lysophospholipid supplementation of pig diets significantly improved the digestibility of dry matter crude protein and energy (Dierick & Decuypere, 2004). Xylanase supplementation of wheat-based broiler feed significantly reduced the *Campylobacter* counts in the caecum to around 10,000 cfu/g but this was not sufficient to improve food safety (Fernandez *et al.*, 2000). Layer hens, which were experimentally infected with *Brachyspira intermedia*, showed reduced faecal excretion of the micro-organism when fed a wheat-based diet supplemented with a commercial enzyme product (Hampson *et al.* 2002). However in subsequent work there was no significant response of feed enzymes in reducing colonization by *B. intermedia* in wheat-based diets. This may have reflected the different enzymes used. In the first trial (Hampson *et al.* 2002) an enzyme mixture containing xylanase and protease was used whereas in the second trial (Phillips *et al.*, 2004), only a xylanase was used.

The proteolytic enzyme, bromelain, which occurs in the pineapple, is recognised as having various systemic effects (Hou *et al.*, 2006). It has been reported to reduce inflammation and blood pressure, regulate the immune system and protect against antimicrobial infections. When rats were feed a diet containing stabilised bromelain for seven days they showed a significant anti-inflammatory response. This was manifested as a reduction in serum cytokines induced by injected lipopolysaccharide (LPS). The anti-inflammatory effect of bromelain was also correlated with reduced LPS-induced nuclear factor kappa B (NF-κB) activity and cyclooxygenase 2 mRNA expression in rat livers. It appears that proteolytic activity of bromelain is required for these systemic effects to be manifested. This offers the intriguing possibility that some feed enzymes may exert an effect on animal health not directly linked to digestion of feed.

Bioactive peptides

Dietary proteins may also play a role in influencing overall metabolism through the concept of bioactive peptides (BAP). These are specific protein fragments from feed ingredients which exert a physiological effect on body function and ultimately influence health. These peptides are inactive within the sequence of the parent protein abut can be released during proteolytic digestion. Both the primary structures and activities of hormone-like peptides have been identified in dietary protein sources (Froetschel, 1996). Both plant and animal protein sources contain BAP. They may exert a number of different activities *in vivo,* affecting the cardiovascular, endocrine, immune and nervous systems as well as various antimicrobial activities (Mine and Kovacs-Nolan, 2006).

Milk and egg proteins in particular have been extensively studied in this regard. Peptides produced by the enzymatic digestion of ovalbumin, one of the major proteins of egg white, were found to be strongly active against *Bacillus subtilis* and to a lesser extent against *Escherichia coli, Bordetella bronchiseptica, Pseudomonas aeruginosa, Serratia maecescens* and *Candida albicans* (Pellegrini *et al.,* 2004). It might at some time be possible to design feeds with particular protein sources that would intrinsically support animal health through the generation of nutricines such as BAP.

Non-digestible oligosaccharides (NDO)

These are often described as prebiotics which are non-digestible feed ingredients that beneficially affect the host animal by selectively stimulating thc growth of desirable bacteria in the large intestine and consequently improve animal health (Gibson and Roberfroid, 1995). Some of these also act as adhesion inhibitors as described above and the precise mode of action of NDOs is difficult to demonstrate.

The NDO, inulin, and lactic acid both gave improved gastrointestinal health in pigs (Pierce *et al.,* 2005). There were improvements in small intestine morphology in the duodenum and the jejunum. However inclusion of both inulin and lactic acid in the diet increased the amounts of of *Lactobacilli* and *Escherichia coli* in the colon. This is clearly not consistent with the concept of NDOs as supporting beneficial bacteria to the detriment of undesirable bacteria. In this study the beneficial effects of inulin on the gastrointestinal health of the pigs was only seen when combined with lactic acid.

Palm kernel meal is also another useful source of NDO with a high content of ß-mannan (Sundu *et al.*, 2006). This ß-mannan has similar properties to yeast cell wall mannan and could also exert immunomodulating activities. It may well be hydrolyzed in the gastrointestinal tract to yield various mannan oligosaccharides.

The effect of NDOs in terms of influencing the microflora in the gastrointestinal tract is not clearly established. Fructose ologosaccharides also showed no effects in modulating the intestinal microflora (Mikkelsen *et al.*, 2003). Whilst the general concept of NDOs as agents for the improvement of animal health is attractive and these materials are safe and easy to use there is more work required to demonstrate how they may be exploited in animal nutrition to positively modulate the gastrointestinal microflora. There is also considerable information published on the effects of NDO as immunomodulators and this is discussed in chapter 6.

Essential oils

There has been considerable work over many years which indicate that various essential oils and some of their constituent components have antimicrobial activities. An extensive study of 66 oils and components identified activities against economically important pathogens such as *Salmonella typhimuirium* DT104, *Escherichia coli* O157:H7 which also had little inhibition towards *Lactobacilli* and *Bifidobacteria* (Gong *et al.*, 2006). The most active compounds were thymol, carvacrol, cinnamon oil, clove oil and eugenol. The compounds tested also retained their efficacy and selectivity against the pathogens tested after incubation with pig caecal digesta. This suggests they may be able to exert an *in vivo* effect but this needs to be established.

Modulation of pathogen virulence

Infectious diseases occur after invasion of the host by a pathogenic micro-organism. However the mere presence of an infectious micro-organism in the body of an animal does not necessarily result in subsequent development of disease. Diet and the nutritional status of the host have an impact upon the degree of virulence of pathogenic micro-organisms.

Nectrotic enteritis and *Clostridia perfringens*

Many clostridial species secrete powerful toxins that cause serious diseases in humans and animals such as tetanus, botulism, gas gangrene and necrotic enteritis. In particular *Clostridia perfringens* is an important pathogen of poultry, and if not controlled, causes necrotic enteritis in chickens, turkeys, and geese (Van Immerseel *et al.*, 2004b, Mcdevitt *et al.*, 2006, Dahiya *et al.*, 2006). The disease syndrome generates lesions in the wall of the small intestine which in turn leads to loss of appetite, the production of dark-coloured faeces, poor growth and increased mortalities.

The acute form of the disease can result in mortalities of broiler flocks of 1% per day for several consecutive days during the last weeks of the rearing period with total mortalities up to 50%. In the subclinical form damage to the intestinal mucosa caused by C. *perfringens* leads to decreased digestion and absorption of nutrients manifested as reduced weight gains and increased feed conversion ratios. Both forms of the disease have serious adverse economic implications for poultry production.

The presence of C. *perfingens* in poultry is also a risk for transmission of the organism to humans through the food chain. Together with *Campylobacter* and *Salmonella*, C. *perfingens* is one of the most frequently isolated foodborne pathogens for humans. Consequently control of necrotic enteritis in poultry has animal production and welfare aspects as well as a food safety aspect. Control of the disease cannot be achieved through the use of antibiotic growth promoters as in the past, and therefore an NbH approach must be developed.

Clostridial bacteria commonly occur in healthy chickens but the pH and high oxygen content of the small intestine do not support extensive growth of the organism and at low population levels the organism is non-pathogenic. For disease symptoms to appear there must be some stress or trigger factor that allows the clostridial bacteria to proliferate and migrate to the lower part of the small intestine. Several stresses which predispose birds to necrotic enteritis are; damage to the intestinal lining by coccidia or by other bacteria, immunosuppression and feed characteristics.

Perhaps the most important predisposing factor is intestinal damage caused by coccidial pathogens. In particular the coccidial species *Eimeria maxima* and *E. acervulina* predispose birds to necrotic enteritis. Removal of coccidiostats from poultry feeds will inevitably lead to increased problems of necrotic enteritis.

Feed composition is also recognised as a strong predisposing factor for necrotic enteritis. Wheat and barley as major raw materials in poultry diets increased the prevalence of necrotic enteritis in broilers compared to the use of maize-based diets (Branton *et al.*, 1987). Use of all wheat in the diet increased mortality attributed to necrotic enteritis, by 6 to 10 times that experienced when only maize was used in the diet (Table 7). Birds that consumed the diet containing approximately equal quantities of wheat and maize exhibited intermediate mortality.

Table 7. Effect of cereal type on performance of broilers at 42 days of age infected with necrotic enteritis.

Cereal	*Weight (kg)*	*FCR*	*Mortality (%)*
Maize	1.749a	1.946a	12/420 (2.9)
Wheat	1.659a	1.861b	101/350 (28.9)
Maize/Wheat	1.757a	1.871b	44/350 (12.6)

Feeds high in barley generated an increased incidence of subclinical necrotic enteritis in broilers compared to those on a maize-based diet (Kaldhusdal and Hofshagen, 1992). The disease was associated with increased feed conversion ratios and retarded growth rates in broilers.

Although there is solid evidence that wheat or barley-based feeds are more prone to encourage the development of necrotic enteritis in poultry than are maize-based diets the precise reasons underlying this is not clear. Branton *et al.* (1996) studied pentosan extracts of wheat and concluded that the water-soluble pentosans of wheat did not directly increase the growth of *C. perfringens*. However there may also be indirect effects of wheat pentosans upon *C. perfringens*. Possibly the pentosans could inhibit other intestinal microflora that naturally controlled the growth of *C. perfingens*. Alternatively the pentosans may directly stimulate intestinal secretions that enhance colonization by *C. perfringens*.

A wide range of dietary factors have been reported to influence the development of necrotic enteritis in poultry (Table 8), (Mcdevitt *et al.*, 2006). In addition to the cereal content of feeds, protein also plays an important role in predisposing birds to necrotic enteritis. Feeds that contain relatively high amounts of proteins or contain poorly digestible proteins will allow proteins to concentrate in the lower portion of the gastrointestinal tract where they will become substrates for growth of the pathogen. The growth of *C.perfingens* is enhanced in a protein-rich environment since it lacks the ability to synthesize 13 out of 20 essential amino acids. Also protein metabolism in the lower part of the gastrointestinal tract will lead to the production of ammonia and amines which will raise the pH of the digesta to a value more conducive to the growth of *C. perfringens*.

Table 8. Dietary components and factors which influence the gastrointestinal tract (GIT) and subsequently the development of necrotic enteritis in poultry.

Dietary component or factor	*Mechanism to promote (+) or to reduce (-) necrotic enteritis*
High levels of wheat and barley	High levels of non-starch polysaccharides; alter viscosity in the GIT. (+)
Types of starches	Resistant starch may become a substrate for the microflora in the GIT. (+)
Protein content and digestibility	Protein concentrates in the GIT and will be a substrate for *C. perfingens*. (+)
Antioxidants	Up-regulates genes associated with the immune response, reduce oxidative damage of the GIT. (-)
Mycotoxins	Damage the GIT, suppress the immune response. (+)
Feed particle size	Influences the physical condition of the GIT and may result in transport of more nutrients to the lower GIT. (+)
Supplementary enzymes	Improve nutrient digestibility and reduce viscosity in the GIT. (-)
Infection with *Eimeria* species	Damages wall of GIT. (+)

Control of necrotic enteritis in poultry production remains an important health issue. In the recent past a useful anti-clostridial agent used in feeds was the antibiotic growth promoter avoparcin but this has now been prohibited from use in the EU. Various medium chain-fatty acids; lauric, myristic, capric, oleic and caprylic acid showed some effect against *C. perfringens in vitro* (Skrivanová *et al.*, 2005). However it is does not necessarily follow that these compounds would have effects *in vivo* and this still needs to be established. A wide range of nutricines such as prebiotics, probiotics, enzymes, essential oils, organic acids and hen egg antibodies have all been used in attempts to reduce the incident of necrotic enteritis in poultry (Dahiya *et al.*, 2006).

There is certainly considerable interest in developing strategies to minimise the stresses on the birds which could predispose them to necrotic enteritis. Moving to a maize-based diet is not possible in many parts of the world and this alleviates but does not control the problem. It is probably important to maintain a healthy, stable gut environment in poultry and to reduce the overall microbial, chemical and physical stress on the birds. Fungal contamination of feeds must be controlled to avoid mycotoxin formation and subsequently immunosuppression. Use of well-stabilised oils and fats in feed manufacture will reduce oxidative stress. Physical consistency of feed characteristics is important so as not to irritate the gut wall.

A major difficulty is studying necrotic enteritis is that in poultry production it tends to be sporadic. This makes it difficult to conduct a series of field trails with putative anti-Clostridial products. It is also very difficult to establish an experimental model to reliably reproduce the disease at the research station level. There still remains a need for an effective nutritional solution to necrotic enteritis in poultry.

Salmonella

A major food borne pathogen is *Salmonella enteric* serovar *enteritidis* which is an invasive *Salmonella* in poultry. The virulence of this invasiveness is controlled by a gene *hilA* and expression of this is decreased by medium-chain fatty acids, caproic, caprylic and capric acids (Van Immerseel *et al.*, 2004a). These medium-chain fatty acids could readily be incorporated into poultry feeds and this could offer some protection against *Salmonella* invasion.

Various non-digestible oligosaccharides reduced the recovery time and improved intestinal function in piglets following infection with *Salmonella typhimurium* (Correa-Matos *et al.*, 2003). Both soyabean oligosaccharides and fructooligosaccharides reduced the virulence of *S.typhimurium* infection associated symptoms. A possible explanation of this reduced virulence is that these non-digestible oligosaccharides were able to generate increased levels of short chain fatty acids; acetic, propionic and butyric, in the colon (Figure 2). These short chain fatty acids are excellent fuels for the cells of the gastrointestinal tract. They promote the development of the digestive and absorptive capacities of the gastrointestinal tract and this probably helps the piglets resist the virulence of *S. typhimurium*.

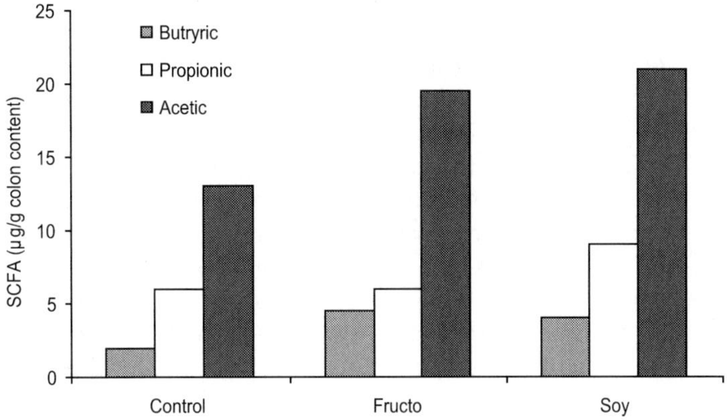

Figure 2. Short chain fatty acids (SCFA) in the colon contents of piglets fed fructooligosaccharides (Fructo) or soyabean oligosaccharides (Soy).

Viruses and antioxidants

Normal cellular metabolism in an animal continuously produces chemical entities that have powerful oxidising properties, known as reactive oxygen species (ROS). The concept of oxidative stress, where antioxidant defences are reduced and ROS accumulate in the body is becoming very important in medical and nutritional research since oxidative stress has been implicated in the pathogenesis of several viral diseases including hepatitis, influenza and AIDS (Beck and Levander, 1998). The ROS are key participants in damage caused by viral infection such as inflammation of epithelial cells in lungs and airways.

Coxsackievirus and myocarditis

Studies on the etiology of Keshan disease in China indicated that both a selenium deficiency and *Coxsackievirus* were necessary components of the disease (Beck *et al.* 1994). Furthermore, the phenotype of the virus was altered in mice suffering from nutritional deficiencies in either vitamin E or selenium such that a non-pathogenic strain of the virus became pathogenic and remained so even when inoculated into nutrient sufficient mice (Table 9), (Beck, 1997).

More detailed work indicated that the change in phenotype of the virus was due to a change in genotype so that it resembled more closely the nucleotide sequence of the virulent strain. Therefore the nutrition of the host had a direct impact in terms of virulence of a potential pathogen which suggests that nutrition is a possible mechanism for driving viral evolution and thus creating altered viruses with different phenotypic properties.

Table 9. Incidence of heart lesions in mice inoculated with a non-pathogenic strain of *Coxsackievirus* recovered from selenium or vitamin E deficient mice.

Diet fed donor mice	*Incidence of heart lesions*
Lard + Se + Vit. E	0/10
Lard – Se + Vit. E	8/10
Lard + Se - Vit. E	9/10

This is quite an alarming scenario since a non-pathogenic virus strain can apparently change into a pathogenic form depending upon the nutrition of the host animal. Furthermore the coxsackievirus is a member of the Picornavirus family, which also includes the virus responsible for Foot and Mouth disease. This demonstrates that the quality of a diet in terms of antioxidant nutricines may contribute to further evolution of new and emerging pathogens.

Oxidative mechanisms have also been shown to be important in the development of influenza in mice (Hennet *et al.*, 1992). Infection of mice with influenza virus resulted in a decrease in the total concentration of the antioxidants glutathione, vitamins C and E in the lungs and liver. In particular changes in the concentrations of antioxidants in the liver were noticed in the early stages of infection. This may reduce the ability of the animals to resist an oxidative stress and the exacerbate the generation of ROS. In addition ROS produced in the lungs may inactivate protease inhibitors which leads to a increase in infectivity of the influenza virus.

Supplementation with excess vitamin E (500ppm for 6 weeks) of old mice reduced influenza lung titers 25-fold when compared with mice fed the control diet (Hayek *et al.*, 1997). Young mice responded less dramatically but five days after infection still showed a 15-fold reduction in virus titers in lung tissue. In this instance high levels of an antioxidant nutricine were able to exert a therapeutic effect to reduce the amount of virus in the tissues.

Newcastle disease virus (NVD) is an important poultry pathogen and the antioxidant BHT has been demonstrated to prevent mortality in chickens exposed to this virus (Brugh, 1977). Inclusion of BHT in poultry diets seems to protect chickens against NVD infection (Brugh, 1984). In a study with purified NVD, BHT caused a 92% reduction in infectivity (Winston *et al.*, 1980). Electron microscopy of the BHT-treated virus particles revealed damage to the envelope of the particle suggesting that BHT may have a direct antiviral effect in this instance.

Iron and infection

Iron is well recognized as an essential element and carries out important functions as a component of oxygen-carrying proteins, haemoglobin and myoglobin. Iron is also a component of many redox enzymes which play an important role in cellular metabolism. Most of the iron in the body is in the haemoglobin of blood erythrocytes and prolonged iron deficiency leads to decreased haemoglobin production and to the onset of anaemia. Conversely excess iron is deposited in tissues and promotes the generation of ROS, which can cause tissue injury and organ failure. Consequently iron absorption and iron tissue levels must be closely regulated to maintain an appropriate iron balance.

Iron status is also important in health maintenance against infectious diseases since invading pathogens must obtain iron for their own metabolic needs. Consequently, although animals have many effective mechanisms of natural resistance to infection, these protective systems only function successfully in an environment where the normal concentration of free iron is virtually zero (Bullen *et al.*, 2005). This low-iron environment is maintained by the activity of hepcidin, which is a peptide hormone (Nemeth and Ganz, 2006) and by the iron binding proteins transferrin and lactoferrin which are normally only 30-40% saturated with iron. Hepcidin controls plasma iron concentration and tissue distribution of iron by inhibiting absorption of iron from the gastrointestinal tract, iron recycling by macrophages, and the mobilization of iron from the liver.

Freely available iron diminishes or destroys normal resistance to infection and increases bacterial virulence. This has been demonstrated with *Vibrio vulnificus* in mice (Wright *et al.*, 1981). The injection of ferric ammonium citrate dramatically reduced the LD50 from 6 x 10^6 to one organism in mice. The replication and virulence of *Mycobacterium tuberculosis* (Cronje *et al.*, 2005) and of *M. bovis* (Denis & Buddle, 2005) was influenced by iron and iron chelating agents. The iron chelator, desferrioxamine, consistently reduced the viability of *M tuberculosis* (Cronje *et al.*, 2005) and addition of lactoferrin to macrophages infected by *M. bovis* blocked replication of the pathogen (Denis & Buddle, 2005). The important pathogen *Campylobacter* has several genes regulating iron acquisition and oxidative stress, which indicates the central role that iron plays in the virulence of this organism (van Vliet *et al.*, 2002). The ability of freely available iron to diminish or destroy normal resistance and to increase bacterial virulence has been demonstrated in at least 18 different bacterial species (Bullen *et al.*, 2005).

Excessive dietary iron induced a normally benign *Coxsackievirus* to damage heart muscle in mice (Beck *et al.*, 2005). High dietary iron gave a similar response to that seen with deficiencies of antioxidants such as vitamin E and selenium (Beck, 1997). The highest heart viral titers were found in mice fed a diet deficient in vitamin E with excess iron which was also the most pro-oxidative diet. However oxidative stress is not the full explanation since the formation of oxidized products, assayed as thiobarbituric acid reactive substances (TBARS), in the liver of the mice did not always correlate with the extent of heart damage.

The control of free iron is important for health maintenance and disease avoidance and organic acids may also play a role here. Many organic acids such as lactic, fumaric and citric acids can form complexes with iron. Phytic acid, which is a common constituent of plant seeds, and therefore also of animal feeds, is a powerful iron chelator. Possible beneficial effect of organic acids in animal nutrition may be related to their antimicrobial activity and their ability to reduce oxidative stress through iron chelation.

Antibiotics and bacterial virulence

There has been considerable debate in the EU over the use of antibiotics in feed as growth promoters, culminating in a total ban of all antibiotic growth promoters in 2006. This was primarily based on the possibility that feeding low levels of antibiotics to animals might develop antibiotic resistance in various bacterial pathogens. In particular there is was concern that enteric bacteria such as *E.coli*, *Salmonella*, and *Campylobacter* with an enhanced antibiotic resistance would transfer from animal to animal or animal to human via the food chain or by direct contact. This could establish a population of virulent bacterial pathogens with antibiotic resistance in both animals and humans (Barton, 2000).

However, concerns about the use of antibiotics in animal production, and the appearance of bacterial resistance is certainly not a new phenomenon and was also expressed quite some time ago (Anderson, 1965). The emergence of ampicillin-resistant *S. typhimurium* strains was traced to the use of this antibiotic to treat or prevent infections in calves. This raised concerns in 1965 that resistant strains of *S.typhimurium* found in calves could transfer resistance to other bacteria such as *E. coli* and subsequently to other human pathogens.

Since that time several other examples of the generation of bacterial resistance to antibiotics have been reported (Witte *et al.*, 2000). Special attention was paid to avoparcin, virginamycin and tylosin because of possible cross-resistance against therapeutic antibiotics used in human medicine. Perhaps the most serious situation was the isolation of glycopeptide-resistant *Enterococcus faecium* in the intestinal flora of animals and humans (Wegener *et al.*, 1999). The antibiotic, avoparcin is also a glycopeptide and consequently animal husbandry came under suspicion as a reservoir of resistant bacteria. Some strains of *Salmonella typhimurium* DT104 have been shown to have resistance against several antibiotics including ampicillin, chloramphenicol, streptomycin, sulfamethoxazole, and tetracycline (Bower and Daeschel, 1999). This multi-resistant strain can thrive in an animal being fed sub-therapeutic doses of antibiotic when competing bacteria from the normal flora are suppressed. An antibiotic stress also induced increased resistance and virulence in the human pathogen *Streptococcus pneumoniae* (Prudhomme *et al.*, 2006). This has implications for the therapeutic use of antibiotics. The application of antibiotics to animals, usually via feed, does obviously pose a risk of developing increased resistance and virulence in pathogenic bacteria.

Conclusions

Enteric diseases which arise when pathogenic microorganisms invade the gastrointestinal tract are a major source of concern in animal production. Therefore an important and basic objective in the development of NbH must be to identify and to exploit various feed raw materials and other bioactive feed ingredients, nutricines, that can inhibit pathogen adhesion, inhibit pathogen growth and ensure that the diet does not increase the virulence of pathogens. Some anti-adhesion factors have been identified such as non-digestible oligosaccharides and tannins. Feed formulation can play a useful role in managing enteric disease. Reduced protein content and the use of cooked rice in piglet diets have given some benefits. Nutricines such as organic acids, enzymes, non-digestible oligosaccharides and esential oils are able to modify the microflora in the gastrointestinal tract with positive health benefits. Feed also influences pathogen virulence, particularly necrotic enteritis in poultry. Good antioxidant status in feeds is beneficial in reducing the pathogenicity of some viruses. Iron status influence the susceptibility of animals to infectious diseases and iron chelators such as deferoxamine or organic acids may play a role here.

References

Adams C. A. (1999) *NUTRICINES Food Components in Health and Nutrition,* Nottingham UK, Nottingham University Press, pp.128.

Adams C. A. (2002) *TOTAL NUTRITION Feeding Animals for Health and Growth,* Nottingham UK, Nottingham University Press, pp. 244.

Anderson, E. S. (1965). Drug resistance and its transfer in *Salmonella typhimurium*. *Nature*, **206**: 579 - 583.

Barton, M. D. (2000). Antibiotic use in animal feed and its impact on human health. *Nutrition Research Reviews*, **13**: 279-299.

Beck, M. A., Kolbeck, P. C., Rohr, L. H., Shi, Q, Morris, V. C. and Levander, O. A. (1994) Increased virulence of a human enterovirus (coxsackievirus B3) in selenium-deficient mice. *Journal of Infectious Diseases*, **170**: 351-357.

Beck, M. A. (1997) Increased virulence of Coxsackievirus B3 in mice due to vitamin E or selenium deficiency. *Journal of Nutrition*, **127**: 966S-970S.

Beck, M. A.; Levander, O. A. (1998). Dietary oxidative stress and the potentiation of viral infection. *Annual Review of Nutrition* **18**: 93-116.

Beck, M. A., Shi, Q., Morris, V. C. and Levander, O. A. (2005). Benign coxsackievirus damages heart muscle in iron-loaded vitamin E-deficient mice. *Free Radical Biology and Medicine*, **38**: 112-116.

Bedford, M. R. (2000). Exogenous enzymes in monogastric nutrition – their current value and future benefits. *Animal Feed Science and Technology*, **86**: 1 - 13.

Bertschinger, H. U., Eggenberger, E., Jucker, H. and Pfirter, H. P (1979). Evaluation of low nutrient, high fibre diets for the prevention of porcine *Escherichia coli* enterotoxaemia. *Veterinary Microbiology*, **3**: 281-290.

Boesen, H. T., Jensen, T. K., Schmidt, A. S., Jensen, B. B., Jensen, S. M. and Moller, K. (2004). The influence of diet on *Lawsonia intracellularis* colonization in pigs upon experimental challenge. *Veterinary Microbiology*, **103**: 35-45.

Bower, C. K. and Daeschel, M. A. (1999). Resistance responses of microorganisms in food environments. *International Journal of Food Microbiology*, **50**: 33-44.

Branton, S. L., Reece F. N. and Hagler Jr., W. M. (1987). Influence of a wheat diet on mortality of broiler chickens associated with necrotic enteritis. *Poultry Science*, **66**: 1326-1330

Branton, S. L., Lott, BB. D., May, J. D., Hedin, P. A., Austin F. W., Latour, M. A. and Day, E. J. (1996). The effects of nonautoclaved and autoclaved water-soluble wheat extracts on the growth of *Clostridium perfringens*. *Poultry Science*, **75**: 335-338

Brugh, M. Jr. (1977). Butylated hydroxytoluene protects chickens exposed to Newcastle disease virus. Science, 197: 1291-1292.

Brugh, M. (1984). Efects of feed additives and feed contaminants on the susceptibility of chickens to viruses. *Progress in Clinical and Biological Research*, **161**: 229-234.

Bullen, J. J., Rogers, H. J., Spalding, P. B. and Ward, C. G. (2005). Iron and infection: the heart of the matter. *FEMS Immunology and Medical Microbiology*, **43**: 325-330.

Byrd, J. A., Anderson, R. C., Callaway, T. R., Moore, R. W., Knape, K. D., Kubena, L. F., Ziprin, R. L. and Nisbet, D. J. (2003). Effect of experimental chlorate product administration in the drinking water on *Salmonella typhimurium* contamination of broiler. *Poultry Science*, **82**: 1403-1406.

Callaway, T. R., Elder, R. O., Keen, J. E., Anderson, R. C. and Nisbet, D. J. (2003). Forage feeding to reduce postharvest *Escherichia coli* populations in cattle, a review. *Journal of Dairy Science*, **86**: 852-860.

Canibe, N., Hojberg, O., Hosgaard, S. and Jensen, B. B. (2005). Feed physical form and formic acid addition to the feed affect the gastrointestinal ecology and growth performance of growing pigs. *Journal of Animal Science*, **83**: 1287-1302.

Cherrington, C. A., Hinton, M. and Chopra, I. (1990). Effect of short-chain organic acids on macromolecular synthesis in *Eschericia coli*. *Journal of Bacteriology,* **68**: 69-74.

Coma, J. (2003). Salmonelaa control in pork: effect of animal nutrition and feeding. *PigNews and Information* **24**: 49N-62N.

Correa-Matos, N. J., Donovan, S. M., Isaacson, R. E., Gaskins, H. R., White, B. A. And Tappenden, K. A. (2003). Fermentable fibre reduces recovery time and improves intestinal function in piglets following *Salmonella typhimurium* infection. *Journal of Nutrition,* **133**: 1845-1852.

Cronje, L., Edmonson, N., Eisenach, K. D. and Bornman, L. (2005). Iron and iron chelating agents modulate *Mycobacterium tuberculosis* growth and monocyte-macrophage viability and effector functions. *FEMS Immunology and Medical Microbiology,* **45**: 103-112.

Dahiya, J. P., Wilkie, D. C., Van Kessel, A. G. and Drew, M. D. (2006). Potential strategies for controlling necrotic enteritis in broiler chickens in post-antibiotic era. *Animal Feed Science and Technology,* **129**: 60-88.

Denis, M. and Buddle, B. M. (2005). Iron modulates the replication of virulent *Mycobacterium bovis* in resting and activated bovine and possum macrophages. *Veterinary Immunology and Immunopathology*, **107**: 189-99.

Dierick, N. A., Decuypere, J., Molly, K. and vanBeek, E. (2002). The combined use of triacylglycerols containing medium-chain fatty acids and exogenous lipolytic enzymes as an alternative for nutritional antibiotics in piglet nutrition. *Livestock Production Science*, **75**: 129-142.

Dierick, N. A. and Decuypere, J. A. (2004). Influence of lipase and/or emulsifier addition on the ileal and faecal nutrient digestibility in growing pigs fed diets containing 4% animal fat. *Journal of the Science of Food and Agriculture*, **84**: 1443-1450.

Edrington, T. S., Callaway, T. R., Anderson, R. C., Genovese, K. J., Jung, Y. S., McReynolds, J. L., Bischoff, K. M., and Nisbet, D. J. (2003). Reduction of *E. coli* O157:H7 populations in sheep by supplementation of an experimental sodium chlorate product. *Small Ruminant Research*, **49**:173-181.

Eklund, T. (1985). The effect of sorbic acid and esters of *p*-hydroxybenzoic acid on the protonmotive force in *Escherichia coli* membrane vesicles. *Journal of General Microbiology*, **131**: 73-76.

Fernandez, F., Sharam, R., Hinton, M. and Bedford, M. R. (2000). Diet influences the colonisation of *Campylobacter jejuni* and the distribution of mucin carbohydrates in the chick intestinal tract.

Cellular and Molecular Life Sciences, **57**: 1793-1801.

Froetschel, M. A. (1996). Bioactive peptides in digesta that regulate gastrointestinal function and intake. *Journal of Animal Science*, **74**: 2500-2508.

Gibson, G. R. and Roberfoid, M. B. (1995). Dietary modulation of the human colonic microbiota. *Journal of Nutrition*, **125**: 1401-1412.

Gong, W. S., Tsao, R., Zhou, T., Yu, H., Poppe, C., Johnson, R. and Du, Z. (2006). Antimicrobial activity of essential oils and structurally related synthetic food additives towards selected pathogenic and beneficial gut bacteria. *Journal of applied Microbiology*, **100**: 296-305.

Hampson, D. J., Phillips, N. D. and Pluske, J. R. (2002). Dietary enzyme and zinc bacitracin reduce colonization of layer hens by the intestinal spirochaete *Brachyspira intermedia*. *Veterinary Microbiology*, **86**: 351-360.

Hayek, M. G., Taylor, S. F., Bender, B. S., Han, S. N., *et al*, (1997). Vitamin E supplementation decreases lung virus titers in mice infected with influenza. *Journal of Infectious Diseases*, **176**: 273-276.

Hennet, T., Peterhans, E. and Stocker, R. (1992). Alterations in antioxidant defences in lungs and liver of mice infected with influenza A virus. *Journal of General Virology*, **73**: 39-46.

Hou, R., C-W., Chen, Y-S., Huang, J-R. and Jeng, K-C. G. (2006). Cross-linked bromelain inhibits lipolysaccharide-induced cytokine production involving cellular signaling suppression in rats. *Journal of Agricultural and Food Chemistry*, **54**: 2193-2198.

Kaldhusdal, M. and Hofshagen, M. (1992). Barley inclusion and avoparcin supplementation in broiler diets 2. Clinical, pathological, and bacteriological findings in a mild form of necrotic enteritis. *Poultry Science*, **71**: 1145-1153.

Lee, C-F., Han, C-K. and Tsau, J-L. (2004). In vitro inhibitory activity of chinese leek extract against *Campylobacter* species. *International Journal of Food Microbiology*, **94**: 169-174.

Leeson, S., Namkung, H., Antongiovanni, M. and Lee, E. H. (2005). Effect of butyric acid on the performance and carcass yield of broiler chickens. *Poultry Science*, **84**: 1418-1422.

Lindecrona, R. H., Jensen, T. K., Jensen, B. B., Leser, T. D., Jiufeng, W. and Møller, K. (2003). The influence of diet on the development of swine dysentry upon experimental infection. *Animal Science*, **76**: 81-87.

Mateos, G. G., Martín F., Latorre, M. A., Vicente, B. and Lázaro, R. (2006). Inclusion of oat hulls in diets for young pigs based on cooked maize or cooked rice. *Animal Science*, **82**: 57-63.

Mcdevitt, R. M., Brooker, J. D., Acamovic, T. and Sparks, N. H. C. (2006). Necrotic enteritis; a continuing challenge for the poultry industry. *World's Poultry Science Journal*, **62**: 221-247.

McDonald, D. E., Pethick, D. W., Pluske, J. R., and Hampson, D. J. (1999). Adverse effects of soluble non-starch polysaccharide (guar gum) on piglet growth and experimental colibacillosis immediately after weaning. *Research in Veterinary Science*, **67**: 245-250.

Mead, G. C. (2002). Factors affecting intestinal colonisation of poultry by campylobacter and role of microflora in control. *World's Poultry Science Journal*, **58**: 169-178.

Mills, A. and Phillips, C. A. (2003). Campylobacter jejuni and the human food chain: a possible source. *Nutrition and Food Science*, **33**: 197-202.

Mikkelsen, L. L., Jakobsen, M. and Jensen, B. B. (2003). Effects of dietary oligosaccharides on microbial diversity and fructoligosaccharide degradiing bacteria in faeces of piglets post-weaning. *Animal Feed Science and Technology*, **109**: 133-150.

Mine Y. and Kovacs-Nolan, J. (2006). New insights in biologically active proteins and peptides derived from hen egg. *World's Poultry Science Journal*, **62**: 87-95.

Montagne, L., Cavaney, F. S., Hampson, D. J., Lallès, J. P. and Pluske, J. R. (2004). Effect of diet composition on postweaning colibacillosis in piglets. *Journal of Animal Science*, **82**: 2364-2374.

Nemeth, E. and Ganz, T. (2006). Regulation of iron metabolism by hepcidin. *Annual Review of Nutrition*, **26**: 323-342.

Nyachoti, C. M., Omogbenigum, F. O., Rademacher, M. and Blank, G. (2006). Performance responses and indicators of gastrointestinal health in early-weaned piglets fed low-protein amino acid-supplemented diets. *Journal of Animal Science*, **84**: 125-134.

Ofek, I., Hasty, D. L., and Sharon, N. (2003). Anti-adhesion therapy of bacterial diseases: prospects and problems. *FEMS Immunology and Medical Microbiology*, **38**: 181-191.

Park, S. F. (2002). The physiology of *Campylobacter* species and its relevance to their role as foodborne pathogens. *International Journal of Food Microbiology*, **74**: 177-188.

Parks, C. W., Grimes, J. L., Ferket, P. R. and Fairchild, A. S. (2001). The effect of mannanoligosaccharides, bambermycins, and virginiamycin on performance of large white male market turkeys. *Poultry Science*, **80**: 718-723.

Partanen, K. H. and Mroz, Z. (1999). Organic acids for performance enhancement in pig diets. *Nutrition Research Reviews*, **12**: 117-145.

Pellegrini, A., Hulsmeier, A., Hunziker, P. and Thomas, U. (2004). Proteolytic fragments of ovalbumin display antimicrobial activity. *Biochimica et Biophysica Acta*, **1672**: 76-85.

Persia; M. E., Young, E. L., Utterback, P. L. and Parsons, C. M. (2006). Effects of dietary ingredients and *Eimeria acervulina* infection on chick performance, apparent metabolizable energy and amino acid digestibility. *Poultry Science*, **85**: 48-55.

Phillips, N. D., La, T., Pluske, J. R. and Hampson, D. J. (2004). A wheat-based diet enhances colonization with the intestinal spirochaete *Brachyspira intermedia* in experimentally infected laying hens. *Avian Pathology*, **33**: 451-457.

Pierce, K. M., Sweeney, T., Brophy, P. O., Callan, J. J., McCarthy, P. and O'Doherty, J. V. (2005). Dietary manipulation post weaning to improve piglet performance and gastro-intestinal health. *Animal Science*, **81**: 347-356.

Pluske, J. R., Siba, P. M., Pethick, D. W., Durmic, Z., Mullan, B. P. and Hampson, D. J. (1996). The incidence of swine-dysentery in pigs can be reduced by feeding diets that limit the amount of fermentable substrate entering the large intestine. *Journal of Nutrition*, **126**: 2920-2933.

Pluske, J. R., Pethick, D. W., Hopwood, D. E. and Hampson, D. J. (2002). Nutritional influences on some major enteric bacterial diseases of pigs. *Nutrition Research Reviews*, **15**: 333-371.

Prudhomme, M., Attaiech, L., Sanchez, G., Martin, B. and Claverys, J-P. (2006). Antibiotic stress induces genetic transformability in the human pathogen *Steptococcus pneumoniae*. *Science*, **313**: 89-92.

Pryde, S. E., Duncan, S. H., Hold, G. L., Stewart, C. S. and Flint, H. J. (2002). The microbiology of butyrate formation in the human colon. *FEMS Microbiology Letters*, **217**: 133-139.

Rhoades, J. R., Gibson, G. R., Formentin, K., Beer, M., Greenberg, N. and Rastall, R. A. (2005). Caseinoglycomacropeptide inhibits adhesion of pathogenic *Escherichia coli* strains to human cells in culture. *Journal of Dairy Science*, **88**: 3455-3459.

Risley, C. R., Kornegay, E. T., Lindemann, M. D. and Weakland, S.M. (1991). Effects of organic acids with or without a microbial culture on performance and gastrointestinal tract measurements of weanling pigs. *Animal Feed Science and Technology,* **35**: 259-270.

Roy, R. D., Edens, F. W., Parkhurst, C. R., Quresh, M. A. and Havenstein, G. B. (2002). Influence of a propionic acid feed additive on performance of turkey poults with experimentally induced poult enteritis and mortality syndrome. *Poultry Science*, **81**: 951-957.

Schwarzer, K. and Adams, C. A. (1996). The influence of specific phospholipids as absorption enhancer in animal nutrition. *Fett/Lipid*, **98**: 304-308.

Shanker, S., Lee, A. and Sorrel, T. C. (1990). Horizontal transmission of *Campylobacter jejuni* amongst broiler chicks: experimental studies. *Epidemiology and Infection*, **104**: 101-110.

Skrivanová, E., Marounek, M., Dlouha, G. and Kanka, J. (2005). Susceptibility of Clostridium perfringens to C_2-C_{18} fatty acids. *Letters in Applied Microbiology*, **41**: 77-

Sundu, B., Kumar, A. and Dingle, J. (2006). Palm kernel meal in broiler diets: effect on chicken performance and health. *World's Poultry Science Journal*, **62**: 316-325.

Tuitoeck, K., Young, L. G., de Lange, C. F. M. and Kerr, B. J. (1997). The effect of reducing excess dietary amino acids on growing-finishing pig performance: An evaluation of the ideal protein concept. *Journal of Animal Science*, **75**: 1575-1583.

Udayamputhoor, R. S., Hariharan, H., Van Lunen, T. A., Lewis, P. J., Heaney, S., Price, L., Woodward, D. (2003). Effects of diet formulations containing proteins from different sources on intestinal colonization by *Campylobacter jejuni* in broiler chickens. *Canadian Journal of Veterinary Research*, **67**: 204-212.

Van Immerseel, F., De Buck, J., Boyen, F., Bohez, L., Pasmans, F., Volf, J., Sevcik, M., Rychlik, I., Hasebrouck, F. and Ducatelle, R. (2004a). Medium-chain fatty acids decrease colonization and invasion through *hilA* suppression shortly after infection of chickens with *Salmonella enterica* serovar enteritidis. *Applied and Environmental Microbiology*, **70**: 3582-3587.

Van Immerseel, F., De Buck, J., Pasmans, F., Huyghebaer, G., Hasebrouck, F. and Ducatelle, R. (2004b). *Clostridium perfringens* in poultry: an emerging threat to animal and public health. *Avian Pathology,* **33**: 537-549

Van Vliet, A. H. M., Ketley, J. M., Park, S. F. and Penn, C. W. (2002). The role of iron in Campylobacter gene regulation, metabolism and oxidative stress. *FEMS Microbiology Reviews*, **26**: 173-186.

Wegener, H. C., Aarestrup, F. M., Jensen, L. B., Hammerum, A. M. and Bager, F. (1999). Use of antimicrobial growth promoters in food animals and *Enterococcus faecium* resistance to therapeutic antimicrobial drugs in Europe. *Emerging Infectious Diseases*, **5**: 329-335.

Whitney, M. H., Shurson, G. C. and Guedes, R. C. (2006). Effect of dietary inclusion of distillers grains with solubles, soybean hulls or a polyclonal antibody product on the ability of growing pigs to resist a *Lawsonia intracellularis* challenge. *Journal of Animal Science*, **84**: 1880-1889.

Winston, V. D., Bolen, J. B. and Consigli, R. A. (1980). Effect of butylated hydroxytoluene on Newcastle disease virus. *American Journal of Veterinary Research*, **41**: 391-394.

Witte, W., Jorsal, S. E., Roth, F. X., Kirchgessner, M., Göransson, L., Lange, S. and Pedersen, K. B. (2000). Future strategies with regard to the use of feed without antibiotics in pig production. *Pig News and Information*, **21**: 27N – 32N.

Wright, A. C., Simpson, L. M. and Oliver, J. D. (1981). Role of iron in the pathogenesis of *Vibrio vulnificus* infections. *Infection and Immunology,* **43**: 503-507.

Xing, J. J., van Heugten, E., Li, D. F., Touchette, K. J., Coalson, J. A., Odgaard, R. L. and Odle, J. (2004). Effects of emulsification, fat encapsulation, and pelleting on weanling pig performance and nutrient digestibiblity. *Journal of Animal Science*, **82**: 2601-2609.

4 Feed-Mycotoxin Interactions

Mycotoxins are potent, toxic molecules, produced as secondary metabolites by moulds contaminating feed raw materials, silages or manufactured animal feeds.(Diaz, 2005, Garon *et al.*, 2006). As they are secondary metabolites, mycotoxins are not essential to mould growth and they are produced sporadically under some sort of stress. They can contaminate a wide variety of feed raw materials such as cereals and oilseeds. They are generally quite heat stable. This was clearly demonstrated by the cooking of Faba beans and wheat contaminated with ochratoxin A. In Faba beans either autoclaved at 115.5°C for two hours or heated at 100°C for six hours ochratoxin A levels were only reduced by 16 and 20% respectively. Cooking of wheat at 100°C for 30 minutes only reduced the ochratoxin A levels by 6% (El-Banna and Scott, 1984). The levels of aflatoxin B_1 in dried wheat were reduced by 50% and by 90% by heating at high temperatures of 150 and 200°C respectively (Hwang and Lee, 2006). Therefore the temperature regimes used in most feed processing conditions are unlikely to have much impact in reducing mycotoxin contamination in feeds. Furthermore the necessity to store feed raw materials in large volumes for substantial periods of time increases the possibility for mould growth and associated mycotoxin production. Consequently mycotoxins are important feed- and food-borne toxic agents as they affect all animal species including avian species, pigs, ruminants, fish and humans (Adams, 2001; Galvano *et al.*, 2005).

Many mycotoxins have damaging cytotoxic properties which seriously affect animal health, manifested as reduced growth performance, immunosuppression or increased mortality. Various common mould species can collectively produce several hundred toxic metabolites with different chemical structures and biological activities. They may be carcinogenic (aflatoxin B_1 and M_1, ochratoxin A, fumonisin B_1), oestrogenic (zearalenone), neurotoxic (fumonisin B_1), nephrotoxic (ochratoxin A, citrinin), dermonecrotic (tricothecenes) or immunosuppressive (aflatoxin B_1, ochratoxin A, and T-2 toxin) (FAO, 2000).

The epithelial cells of the gastrointestinal tract are likely to be the first body cells to be exposed to mycotoxins and several mycotoxins can cause damage to the cells of the gastrointestinal tract. For example in dogs, chickens and pigs ochratoxin A causes necrosis of the mucosa of the gastrointestinal tract (Bouhet and Oswald, 2005). Similarly the ingestion of patulin-contaminated feed leads to gastrointestinal injury including ulceration and inflammation of the stomach and intestines. Exposure to deoxynivalenol (DON) and T-2 toxin is responsible for vomiting, diarrhoea, and malabsorption of nutrients. Fumonisin B_1 has been associated with diarrhoea in laying hens and day–old cockerels.

Symptoms of mycotoxin toxicity

Increased organ weight

A common effect of mycotoxicosis the enlargement of organ size as a proportion of body weight. Ochratoxin A increased the relative weights of liver, kidney, gizzard and spleen in broilers (Elissalde *et. al.*, 1994). A similar response was seen in an experiment with aflatoxin in broilers where liver and gizzard weights were quite significantly increased by 400 ppb of aflatoxin in the feed (Swamy and Devegowda, 1998). The toxicity of cyclopiazonic acid was also expressed through increased relative organ weights (Dwyer *et al.*, 1997) (Table 1).

A somewhat similar response was seen in pigs fed deoxynivalenol (DON) from contaminated wheat for seven weeks where liver and kidney weights increased (Trenholm *et al.*, 1994).

Table 1. Relative organ weights (% of body weight) of broilers fed different levels of ochratoxin A, aflatoxin B_1 and cyclopiazonic acid.

Ochratoxin A (mg/kg)	*Relative liver weight (%)*	*Relative gizzard weight (%)*	*Relative kidney weight (%)*
0	3.28	2.51	0.56
3	4.25	3.17	0.78
Aflatoxin (mg/kg)			
0	2.21	1.89	
0.1	2.27	2.02	
0.2	2.33	2.11	
0.4	2.96	2.43	
Cyclopiazonic acid (mg/kg)			
0		2.61	0.463
45		2.99	0.521

However the response of organ weights to mycotoxins has not been consistent. Pigs fed on *Fusarium* contaminated grains showed a reduction in both relative and absolute liver and kidney weights (Swamy *et al.*, 2002). In this later study the reduced liver and kidney weights were ascribed to the combined results of feed refusal and systemic toxicity of *Fusarium* mycotoxins. Broiler breeders fed grains contaminated with *Fusarium* mycotoxins also did not show any increases in the relative weights of liver, spleen or kidney (Yegani *et al.*, 2006). Possibly increased organ weight is not symptomatic of toxicity due to *Fusarium* mycotoxins.

Immunosuppression

Many mycotoxins are known to alter the immune function in animals frequently causing immunosuppression.

Aflatoxin is an immunomodulating agent that acts primarily on cell-mediated immunity and phagocytic cell function rather than on adaptive immunity. There is considerable evidence of the immunosuppressive effects of aflatoxins in poultry, pigs and rats (Bondy and Pestka, 2000). Moreover when aflatoxins were administered to broiler hens or sows the progeny, chicks and piglets, also showed effects of the aflatoxin in terms of immunosuppression. It is well known that aflatoxin in feeds of lactating animals can be transferred into milk and hence the stringent controls on aflatoxin levels in feeds and feed ingredients.

Fumonisins are produced primarily by the fungi *Fusarium verticilloides* and *F. proliferatum* and have an apparent species specificity in terms of toxicity. Purified fumonisin B_1 causes leukoencephalomalacia in horses and pulmonary oedema in pigs. In mice it affects the liver whereas in rats the primary target is the kidneys. However fumonisins also have a general effect upon the immune system that is not species specific. Poultry are relatively resistant to the effects of fumonisisn and show few signs of toxicity after consuming contaminated feed (Yegani *et al.*, 2006). However these mycotoxins also affect the immune system in poultry manifested as depressed thymus weights and depressed antibody responses (Li *et al.*, 2000a; Li *et al.*, 2000b).

Ochratoxin A is a potent kidney toxin in poultry and pigs and has wide ranging immunosuppressive effects in pigs, poultry and rodents.

Tricothecenes are a large group of mycotoxins which include deoxynivalenol (DON) and T-2 toxin as the most common examples. Experimental acute oral exposure to tricothecene mycotoxins causes severe damage to actively dividing cells in bone marrow, lymph nodes, spleen, thymus and intestinal mucosa. One of the most dramatic effects of DON is a pronounced elevation in serum immunoglobulin A (IgA) and a concurrent depression in IgM and IgG. It seems that the immune system is a major target for the tricothecenes.

An important consequence of mycotoxins suppressing the immune system is also manifested in reduced response to vaccination. Layer-breeders given a single vaccination against Newcastle disease and fed a diet containing 500 ppb of aflatoxin showed a significant decrease in haemagglutination-inhibition titers (Boulton *et al.*, 1980).

The immunosuppressive effect of various mycotoxins will increase the susceptibility of the animals to opportunistic infections from pathogens present in commercial livestock production systems (CAST-Report, 2003). This has been well demonstrated by the effects of ochratoxin A together with *Salmonella* in broiler chicks (Elissalde *et al.,* 1994). At 21 days there was almost a three-fold increase in mortality of chicks infected with *S. typhimurium* and also given ochratoxin A in the feed compared to chicks only infected with *Salmonella* (Table 2). Chicks at this age would normally not be particularly sensitive to *Salmonella* but the presence of the mycotoxin probably suppressed the immune system of the broiler chicks and they become more sensitive to pathogenic bacteria.

Table 2. Effect of ochratoxin A and *Salmonella typhimurium* on broiler performance over 21 days.

Treatment		*Performance characteristics*	
Ochratoxin A (3 mg/kg)	*Salmonella (100 million cfu)*	*Weight gain (g)*	*Mortality (%)*
-	-	640	0
+	-	395	0
-	+	545	4.5
+	+	325	13.2

Ochratoxin A also exacerbated the effects of *Salmonella gallinarum* in broilers (Gupta et al., 2005). Birds infected with *S. gallinarum* in the absence of ochratoxin A had 11.5% mortality and this more than doubled to 28.8% in the presence of ochratoxin A.

A similar response was seen with ochratoxin A and *Escherichia coli* in broiler chicks (Kumar *et al.*, 2003). The presence of Ochratoxin A in poultry rations increased the mortality and the severity of *E. coli* infections. Mortality was 14.3% in chicks infected with *E. coli* but not given ochratoxin A. Chicks fed ochratoxin A and infected with *E. coli* showed a greatly increased mortality rate of 37.5%.

The immunomodulatory interactions of mycotoxins and infectious pathogens is an important aspect of animal production. It would be very useful if nutritional regimes could be devised that would protect livestock from the immunosuppressive effects of mycotoxins. For example the carotenoid lutein and some non-digestible oligosacharides have recognised immunostimulating effects and their interaction with mycotoxins would be of interest.

Oxidative stress

Mycotoxins can also be a source of oxidative stress and contribute to the development of a range of non-infectious diseases. Feeding low levels of ochratoxin A (1 ppm) to rats resulted in a 22% decrease in alpha-tocopherol levels in the blood plasma and to a five-fold increase in the expression of the oxidative stress responsive protein, haem oxygenase-1 in the kidney (Gautier *et al.*, 2001). This strongly suggests that ochratoxin A evokes an oxidative stress, which may contribute at least in part to ochratoxin A renal toxicity and carcinogenicity.

Mycotoxins and legislation

Mycotoxin-producing moulds grow on staple raw materials used for animal feeds and for human foods. Therefore mycotoxins must be considered persistent and common contaminants of feed and foods. Since both the animal and human populations are affected by the presence of mycotoxins, they present a public health problem of major concern world-wide. Extreme vigilance and careful management of feed and food is vital to ensure that levels of mycotoxins are kept acceptably low.

Because of the risks of food-borne mycotoxins to the health of animals and humans it is not surprising that many countries have instituted regulations to control the maximum amount of mycotoxins that can be accepted in feed raw materials and animal feeds. In most cases this control only applies to one toxin, aflatoxin and strict EU regulations exist to cover possible aflatoxin contamination as illustrated in Table. 3.

Table 3. Aflatoxin B_1 content of feedstuffs permitted in the European Union.

Feedingstuff	*Maximum Aflatoxin B_1 Content (mg/kg)*
Raw materials	0.02
Complete feeds for cattle, sheep and goats excepting:	0.02
Complete dairy feeds	0.005
Complete feeds for calves and lambs	0.01
Complete feeds for pigs and poultry (excepting young animals)	0.02
Other complete feeds	0.01
Supplementary feeds for cattle, sheep and goats (excepting supplementary feeds for dairy cows, calves and lambs).	0.02
Supplementary feeds for pigs and poultry (excepting young animals)	0.02
Other supplementary feeds	0.005

The EU is in the process of establishing guidance values for other mycotoxins in feeedstuffs as shown in Table 4. These mycotoxins do not accumulate to any significant extent in animal products such as meat or milk, so the limits are based on requirements for animal welfare. Susceptibility varies between species, but pigs are in general the most

Table 4. Some guidance values for mycotoxins proposed by the EU in animal feed materials.

Mycotoxin	*Feed Material*	*Guidance value (mg/kg)*
Deoxynivalenol (DON)	Cereals and cereal products with the exception of maize by-products	8.00
	Maize by-products	12.00
	Complementary and complete feedingstuffs with the exception of:	5.00
	Complementary and complete feedingstuffs for pigs:	0.90
	Complementary and complete feedingstuffs for calves (<4 months), lambs and kids	2.00
Zearalenone	Cereals and cereal products with the exception of maize by-products	2.00
	Maize by-products	3.00
	Complementary and complete feedingstuffs for piglets and gilts (young sows)	0.10
	Complementary and complete feedingstuffs for sows and fattening pigs	0.25
	Complementary and complete feedingstuffs for calves, dairy cattle, sheep, (including lamb) and goats (including kids)	0.50
Fumonisins B_1 and B_2	Maize and maize products	60.00
	Complementary and complete feedingstuffs for:	
	Pigs, horses, rabbits and pet animals	5.00
	Fish	10.00
	Poultry, calves (<4 months), lambs and kids	20.00
	Adult animals (>4 months) and mink	50.00
Ochratoxin A	Cereals and cereal products)	0.25
	Complementary and complete feedingstuffs for pig	0.05
	Complementary and complete feedingstuffs for poultry	0.10

sensitive species and so the recommended levels are lower for materials used in diets for pigs than in diets for other species.

Due to the wide range of mycotoxins that can contaminate animal feeds and their variable chemical composition, protection against mycotoxins is a relatively difficult task. There are currently three nutritional solutions to deal with mycotoxins. Firstly, mould growth in feed raw materials and in feeds should be minimised so that the prevalence and growth of toxigenic moulds is reduced. Secondly, mycotoxin-binding nutricines can be incorporated into feeds to reduce the absorption of the toxins into the body of the animal. Thirdly, dietary interventions may reduce the toxic effects of mycotoxins.

Control of mycotoxins

Prevent mould growth

Cereal grains can be initially contaminated by so-called "field moulds" such as, *Alternaria, Cladosporium* and *Fusarium,* whilst developing on the plants in the field. Field moulds require high relative humidities and water contents, typically 20-21%, and are not able to compete in drier storage conditions. Stored grain becomes dominated by species of "storage moulds" such as, *Aspergillus, Monascus, Mucor, Penicillium,* and *Wallemia* which can grow at moisture contents from 13-18%. These various mould species can collectively produce several hundred toxic metabolites, and the major contaminants of feed raw materials are listed in Table 5.

Table 5. Major mycotoxins found in feed raw materials.

Mycotoxin	*Fungal strain*
Aflatoxins,	*Aspergillus* spp.
Fumonisins	*Fusarium moniliforme*
Ochratoxin A	*Aspergillus* and *Penicillium* spp.
Tricothecenes	Several mould spp.
Zearalenone	*Fusarium* spp.

Mycotoxins may not necessarily occur in feeds one at a time since many fungal species are capable of simultaneously producing several mycotoxins (Bottalico, 1998). It is therefore highly likely that mould contamination of feeds would lead to the production of several mycotoxins. Furthermore there is considerable evidence that multiple mycotoxins cause serious disease syndromes in animals raised for food (Kubena *et al.,* 1989, 1997).

Feeding mouldy grain will generally lead to poor animal productivity as a consequence of the various mycotoxins which could be produced. This is illustrated in laying hens (Garaleviciene *et al.*, 2000), (Table 6). At the end of this trial body weight was 3-4% lower and feed intake was 10% and 34% lower in hens consuming mouldy barley, compared to control birds fed mould-free barley. Egg production was also reduced, as was dry matter and crude protein digestibility. The mouldy barley contained ergosterol, ochratoxin A, zearalenone, and nivalenol which is a good demonstration of the complex mycotoxin patterns likely to be found in nature.

Table 6. The effect of moulded barley on the performance of laying hens.

Performance parameter	*Feed*		
	Mould-free barley	*Moulded barley (1997)*	*Moulded barley (1998)*
Initial liveweight (32 weeks)	1676	1673	1678
Final liveweight (39 weeks)	1688	1619	1606
Feed intake (g/day)	142.2	127.5	94.4
FCR (g feed/g egg)	2.82	2.86	3.33
Egg production (g/day)	50.5	44.5	28.0

Since mycotoxins only occur if there has first been mould contamination of raw materials or feeds, the first line of defence is clearly to reduce mould growth to the minimum. During harvest it is important to prevent excessive damage to kernels, which may predispose them to infection during storage. Mould infections and subsequent mycotoxin production can be reduced by careful harvesting of cereal crops. Thus harvesting at the appropriate date, with suitable equipment and careful harvesting procedures to minimize crop damage, as well as the removal of damaged portions of crops and high moisture plant parts is an important first step to obtain good quality feed raw materials.

There are several important parameters which promote mould growth (Nahm, 1990). If moisture levels exceed 13-14% or the relative humidity exceeds 80-85% moulds are likely to grow. When temperatures rise above 50°C moulds grow very rapidly. Cooler temperatures retard mould growth but do not completely inhibit it. Damaged and broken grains open areas for mould growth in stored cereals or feeds. Insect infestation is frequently associated with mould growth.

Dried feed raw materials stored with no condensation or re-wetting in the silos can remain in good condition for a long time. However this is frequently impractical and in many raw material transactions there is no financial premium for excessively dry materials. Drying of raw materials is also a costly exercise.

The judicious use of organic-acid based mould inhibitors can prevent excessive mould contamination and reduce existing mould levels. This can be very important in raw materials that are stored for some time. The most effective products need to be based on propionic acid. Formic acid is not as inhibitory to mould growth as is propionic acid and may allow aflatoxin production in stored materials (Holmberg *et al.*, 1989). Inoculation of moist barley with *Aspergillus parasiticus* and treatment of the barley with formic acid (5kg/tonne) promoted the development of aflatoxin above the control, whereas treatment with propionic acid (3 kg/tonne) completely inhibited mycotoxin production. Many proprietary mould inhibitors based on propionic acid and its salts are available and effectively reduce mould contamination in feeds.

As an extra precaution empty silos can be dusted with mould inhibitors before fresh grain or feed is loaded into them and this will help to keep the grain or feed storage and delivery systems free from build-up of moulds. Storage of harvested crops without delay, in hygienic storage facilities under moisture-, temperature-, humidity- and insect-control and the addition of antifungal agents will diminish fungal growth.

Treatment of feed for piglets with a proprietary mould inhibitor gave useful improvements in total weight gain, daily feed intake and feed to gain ratio compared to a control untreated feed, (Table 7), (Rahnema and Neal, 1994). Piglets consuming feed treated with a mould inhibitor consumed 5.9% more feed than piglets on the control diet which gave an increase in total weight of 10.58% over the control.

Table 7. Effect of liquid mould inhibitor on growth performance of weaned piglets (averages per pen).

Growth characteristic	*Treatment*	
	Control	*Mould inhibitor (1 kg/tonne)*
Total weight gain (kg)	107.33	118.69
Average daily gain (kg)	5.11	5.65
Daily feed intake (kg)	9.44	10.00
Feed/Gain	1.85	1.77

Although the use of organic acid-based mould inhibitors can reduce the amount of mould growth and therefore subsequent mycotoxin production it does not influence the mycotoxins that may have been produced earlier. These toxic compounds are very stable and will remain in the infected commodity even if no further mould growth can be seen or detected.

Prevention of fungal infections during plant growth, harvest, storage and distribution would be the most rational and efficient way to avoid mycotoxins in feed raw materials and in feeds and thus avoid their negative impacts. However the complex processes involved in mycotoxin production by moulds make it difficult to predict which toxin will be produced, when it will be produced and in what concentration. Furthermore mycotoxins in general are quite stable substances, which can persist for a long time in stored materials and which will survive feed processing conditions. Unfortunately it is not possible to prevent entirely the production of mycotoxins before the harvest of agricultural crops, in storage, or during processing operations. Therefore contamination of grains with mycotoxins will frequently occur despite the most strenuous efforts of prevention and these may have serious health and economic impacts. Unfortunately there are no physical or chemical treatments available which are simple and economically feasible to decontaminate feeds.

Mycotoxin inactivation

The second strategy to mitigate the adverse effects of mycotoxins is to incorporate mycotoxin inactivators into the feeds. This strategy is simple in practice and has been the subject of considerable research in recent years (Doll and Danicke, 2004). The mode of action of mycotoxin inactivating products is generally based on the adsorption of mycotoxins onto nutritionally inert materials which should have the capacity to specifically and tightly bind and immobilize mycotoxins present in feed. This will prevent, or at least limit absorption, of mycotoxins from the gastrointestinal tract into the body of the animal. An ideal mycotoxin binder would be able to bind several different mycotoxins as feeds are frequently contaminated with more than one mycotoxin. Such products also should not bind vitamins, minerals or other nutrients and render them non-available to the animal.

Various absorbing materials which have been used include; charcoal, zeolites, bentonite, spent bleaching clay from vegetable oil refining, hydrated sodium calcium aluminosilicate, acidic phyllosilicate, products derived from yeast, cholestyramine anion exchange resin and humic acid (Avantaggiato *et al.*, 2005; Bailey *et al.*, 1998; Dwyer *et al.*, 1997; Jansen van Rensburg *et al.*, 2006; Ramos and Hernandéz, 1997; Schell *et al.*, 1993). The main problem is that mycotoxins are chemically quite diverse and so no single toxin-binding compound is likely to be effective for all mycotoxins. The largest and most complex class of mycotoxin binding agents are various silicate minerals. This includes clay minerals in the groups of such as montmorillonite/smectite, kaolinite, bentonite and illite. There has also been considerable work conducted on yeast cell-wall products as mycotoxin binders. .

A major obstacle in the evaluation of mycotoxin binding products is related to the inadequacy of *in vitro* models in predicting responses in the animal (Diaz and Smith, 2005). Nevertheless *in vitro* models are extremely useful in identifying putative mycotoxin binding agents. If an experimental mycotoxin binding agent cannot bind mycotoxins *in vitro* there is little likelihood that it will do so *in vivo*.

A laboratory model that mimics the metabolic processes of the gastrointestinal tract of healthy pigs has been used to study intestinal absorption of mycotoxins from contaminated feed (Avantaggiato *et al.*, 2003). In this system there was a significant reduction in the intestinal absorption of zearalenone released from contaminated wheat with the inclusion of activated charcoal or cholestyramine as binding agents. When 2% of activated charcoal or cholestyramine was added to the model system the gastrointestinal absorption of zearalenone was reduced from 32% to 5%and 16% respectively. In practical animal nutrition neither of these binding agents are likely to be used. Activated charcoal in particular is a very powerful adsorbing agent and would probably adsorb nutrients as well as mycotoxins. Nevertheless the gastrointestinal model system is a rapid and physiologically relevant method to test the efficacy of adsorbent materials to bind mycotoxins. This would make it a useful preliminary screening test. However, it is also extremely important that any *in vitro* results be supported by *in vivo* experiments utilising the species for which the product is intended.

Humic acid was able to bind aflatoxin B_1 with high affinity *in vitro* (Jansen van Rensburg *et al.*, 2006). In broilers the humic acid product could alleviate some of the toxic effects of aflatoxins such as avoiding liver damage and stomach and heart enlargement but a yeast cell wall product was not effective here.

A glucomannan preparation from yeast was able to prevent some of the adverse effects of *Fusarium* mycotoxins in broiler breeders (Yegani *et al.*, 2006). The feeding of contaminated diets decreased antibody titers against infectious bronchitis virus and this was prevented by the yeast product. However in this trial the mycotoxins did not influence feed consumption nor body weight.

Dietary interventions to reduce the effect of mycotoxins

The complete elimination of mycotoxins present in animal feeds either through mould inhibition or by the use of mycotoxin binders will not always be completely successful. Therefore the third strategy to minimise mycotoxin problems is the use of various dietary interventions to ameliorate the effects of mycotoxins in the animal that has consumed contaminated feed.

Microorganisms in the gastrointestinal tract of animals are an important detoxifying system for the animal. This is probably the reason that ruminants are more resistant to the effects of mycotoxins than monogastric animals as the toxins may be metabolized by the rumen microorganisms. The development of nutritional programmes to promote the activity of microorganisms able to degrade mycotoxins in the gastrointestinal tract could be a useful research topic.

There is already some evidence that components of feed may be beneficial in ameliorating the effects of mycotoxins. Protein, or the amino acid cysteine supplementation, assists the biochemical detoxification of aflatoxin and alleviates some of the adverse effects in the animal. This may be due to the activity of a glutathione (GSH) detoxification system in the liver. Glutathione is a tripeptide which contains cysteine and it binds aflatoxin in the liver and renders it non-toxic after which it is excreted in the bile, and subsequently passes into the urine.

The involvement of GSH in mycotoxin protection suggests that at least some toxic effects of mycotoxins may be due to an oxidative stress. This was further studied in work with rats dosed with DON and T-2 mycotoxins (Rizzo *et al.*, 1994). If the feeds were also deficient in the antioxidants selenium, ascorbic acid and α-tocopherol there were increases in lipid peroxidation of 21% and 268% observed in rats which were administered DON and T-2 toxin respectively, compared to rats receiving diets adequate in antioxidants. It appears that these tricothecene mycotoxins stimulate lipid peroxidation in the livers of rats deficient in antioxidants.

One mode of action of the toxicity of ochratoxin A is the generation of lipid peroxides in both rats and chicks which leads to tissue damage (Hoehler *et al.*, 1997). Further work with rats indicated that ochratoxin A caused a 22% decrease in α-tocopherol blood plasma levels and a five –fold increase in the oxidative stress protein haem oxygenase-1 specifically in the kidney (Gautier *et al.*, 2001). The antioxidant α-tocopherol exerted a protective effect against ochratoxin A in a susceptible bovine mammary cell culture (Baldi *et al.*, 2004). These results strongly suggest that nutritional supplementation with antioxidants can counteract short term toxicity of ochratoxin A

Antioxidants BHA and BHT inhibit aflatoxin carcinogenesis in animals. Treatment of rats with BHA greatly reduced the liver carcinogenic effect of aflatoxin (Monroe *et al.*, 1986). The production of protective enzymes were induced by BHA which increased the biliary excretion of an aflatoxin glutathione conjugate so less aflatoxin was left in the liver and more was excreted in the urine (Table 8). The binding of aflatoxin to liver DNA was also greatly reduced by BHA which is important in the liver carcinogenic effect of aflatoxin.

Turkeys are extremely sensitive to the adverse effects of aflatoxin B_1 which is due to a combination of the efficient activation of aflatoxin by cytochrome P450 and a deficient detoxification by glutathionine S-transferases (Klein et al., 2003). Supplementation of turkey feeds with the antioxidant, BHT, prevented the toxic effects of aflatoxin B_1 ((Klein et al., 2003; Coulombe et al., 2005). The mechanism of protection was primarily through inhibition of enzymatic activation of aflatoxin in the liver. At the same time this antioxidant substantially increases the activities and expression of phase II enzymes known to be important in the detoxification of aflatoxin B_1. Rather high levels of BHT of 4 kg/tonne were utilized which would have serious practical implications.

Table 8. Distribution of aflatoxin in the rat 2 hours after dosing.

Treatment	*Liver (% of dose)*	*Urine (% of dose)*
Control	18.2	0.35
BHA	9.6	3.03

In broilers fed aflatoxin contaminated feed, BHT alleviated the adverse effects of the mycotoxin on weight gain and feed efficiency (Ehrich et al., 1986). By contrast ethoxyquin was ineffective in protecting chicks from the effects of aflatoxin in the feed even though it is a well-recognised feed antioxidant. Unlike BHT, ethoxyquin was unable to induce the activities of chick liver enzymes that detoxify aflatoxin.

Administration of N-acetylcysteine, an acetylated derivative of the amino acid cysteine, prevented the adverse effects of aflatoxin toxicity on weight gain and FCR. It also diminished the severity of histological lesions in liver and kidney of broilers (Valdivia et al., 2001).

N-acetyl cysteine has been widely prescribed to humans in several countries and its safety and pharmacological properties are well established. It is an excellent source of sulfhydryl groups and is capable of stimulating synthesis of glutathione which is also probably involved in reducing the effects of mycotoxins. N-acetyl cysteine may be a very useful compound to control aflatoxicosis in broilers and could be useful on its own or combined with a toxin-binding product.

A glucomannanoligosaccharide present in the cell walls of *Saccharomyces cerevisiae* has been reported to exert a beneficial effect against aflatoxins in broiler feed (Swamy and Devegowda, 1998). Supplementation of feed contaminated with aflaltoxin by the glucomannanoligosaccharide showed some improvements in body weight and feed efficiency but these did not return to the level seen when feed without aflatoxin was used. Also titres against Newcastle Disease and Infectious Bursal Disease were improved by including the glucomannanoligosaccharide in feeds that contained aflatoxin but again remained significantly below the values seen in birds fed aflatoxin-free feed. The possible mode of action maybe some degree of immunostimulation but it could not completely overcome the negative effects of aflatoxin on bird performance. Beta-glucans from yeast cell walls are already used in aquaculture as immunostimulants and have also been shown to up-regulate the innate immunes response in immature chickens against *Salmonella* (Lowry *et al.*, 2005).

In pigs consuming feed containing *Fusarium* mycotoxins incorporation of a glucomannanoligosaccharide was unable to overcome the adverse effects of reduced feed intake and reduced weight gain (Swamy *et al.*, 2002). However the supplementation of 0.2% of the glucomannan-oligosaccharide was effective in preventing some neurochemical changes occasioned by the feeding of mycotoxin-contaminated diets.

Pig feeds contaminated with *Fusarium* mycotoxins can have toxic effects upon the foetuses near the end of gestation and result in increased stillbirths with a concomitant reduction in the number of piglets born alive (Table 9) (Díaz-Llano and Smith, 2006). This effect was reduced by including a glucomannanoligosaccharide in the feed at 0.2%.

Table 9. The influence of *Fusarium* mycotoxins on the reproductive performance of gilts.

Reproductive	*Treatment*		
performance	*Control*	*Contaminated*	*Contaminated +GMO*
Total piglets born per litter	9.8	10.0	10.8
Stillbirths (%)	6.3	15.5	4.6
Born alive (%)	90.5	80.7	95.4

GMO: glucomannanoligosaccharide from yeast

Conclusions

Mycotoxin contamination of feed raw materials and feeds is probably an inevitable event in animal production. Management and control of mycotoxins however is technically well-established. Precautions can be taken at time of harvest and during the storage of raw materials to reduce or avoid mould contamination. Mycotoxin binding products can be incorporated into feeds to reduce the absorption of mycotoxins from the gastrointestinal tract. Lastly various dietary interventions can be utilized to minimise the effect of mycotoxins on animal growth and health.. Management of mycotoxins will become a very important part of NbH, particularly since mycotoxins pose a threat to the immune system of animals and a strategy of health maintenance and disease avoidance must ensure that animals have an optimum immune system.

References

Adams, C. A. Virtues of Cleanliness: Feed quality and Hygiene *in* TOTAL NUTRITION Feeding Animals for Health and Growth. Nottingham

University Press, Nottingham, UK (2001) pp. 21-45.
Avantaggiato, G., Havenaar, R. and Visconti, A. (2003). Assessing the zearalenone-binding activity of adsorbent materials during passage through a dynamic in vitro gastrointestinal model. Food and Chemical Toxicology, 41: 1283-1290.

Avantaggiato, G., Solfrizzo, M. and Visconti, A. (2005). Recent advances on the use of adsorbent materials for detoxification of *Fusarium* mycotoxins. Food Additives and Contaminants, 22: 379-388.

Bailey, R. H., Kubena, L. F., Harvey, R. B., Buckley, S. A. and Rottinghaus, G. E. (1998) Efficacy of various inorganic sorbents to reduce the toxicity of aflatoxin and T-2 toxin in broiler chickens. Poultry Science, 77: 1623-1630.

Boulton, S. L., Dick, J. W. and Hughes, B. L. (1980). Effects of dietary aflatoxin and ammonia-inactivated aflatoxin on Newcastle disease antibody titers in layer-breeders. Avian Diseases, 26: 1-6.

Baldi, A., Losio, M. N., Cheli, F., Rebucci, R., Sangalli, L., Fusi, E., Bertasi, B., Pavoni, E., Carli, S. and Politis, I. (2004). Evaluation of the protective effects of a-tocopherol and retinol against ochratoxin A cytotoxicity. British Journal of Nutrition, 91: 507-512.

Bondy, G. and Pestka, J. J. (2000). Immunomodulation by fungal toxins. Journal of Toxicology and Environmental Health, Part B, 3: 109-143.

Bottalico A., 1998. Review: Fusarium diseases of cereals: species complex and related mycotoxin profiles in Europe. Journal of Plant Pathology 80: 85-103.

Bouhet, S. and Oswald, I. P. (2005). The effects of mycotoxins, fungal food contaminants, on the intestinal epithelial cell-derived innate immune response. Veterinary Immunology and Immunopathology, 108: 199-209.

CAST Report, (2003). Mycotoxins, Risks in Plant, Animal and Human Systems. Task Force Report 139, Council of Agricultural Science and Technology, Ames Iowa. pp 81.

Coulombe, R. A., Guarisco, J. A., Klein, P. J. and Hall, J. O. (2005). Chemoprevention of aflatoxicosis in poultry by dietary butylated hydroxytoluene. Animal Feed Science and Technology, 121: 217-225

Diaz, D. E. (2005) *ed*: The Mycotoxin Blue Book. Nottingham University Press, Nottingham, UK pp.349.

Diaz, D. E. and Smith, T. K. (2005). Mycotoxin sequestering agents: practical tools for the neutralisation of mycotoxins. *In*: The Mycotoxin Blue Book. *Ed:* D. E. Diaz. Nottingham University Press, Nottingham, UK pp.323-339.

Díaz-Llano, G. and Smith, T. K. (2006). Effects of feeding grains naturally contaminated with *Fusarium* mycotoxins with and without a polymeric glucomannan mycotoxin adsorbent on reproductive performance and serum chemistry of pregnant gilts. Journal of Animal Science, 84: 2361-2366.

Doll, S. and Danicke, S. (2004). In vivo detoxification of *Fusarium* toxins. Archives of Animal Nutrition, 58: 419-441.

Dwyer, M. R., Kubena, L. F., Harvey, R. B., Mayura, K., Sarr, A. B., Buckley, S., Bailey, R. H. and Phillips, T. D. (1997). Effects of inorganic adsorbents and cyclopiazonic acid in broiler chickens. Poultry Science, 76: 1141-1149.

Ehrich, M., Driscoll, C. and Larsen, C. (1986). Ability of ethoxyquin and butylated hydroxytoluene to counteract deleterious effects of dietary aflatoxin in chicks. Avian Diseases, 30: 802-806.

El-Banna, A. A. and Scott, P. M. (1984). Fate of mycotoxins during processing of foodstuffs III. Ochratoxin A during cooking of Faba beans (*Vicia faba*) and polished wheat. Journal of Food Protection, 47: 189-192.

Elissalde, M. H., Ziprin, R. L., Huff, W. E., Kubena, L. F. and Harvey, R. B. (1994). Effect of ochratoxin A on *salmonella*-challenged broiler chicks. Poultry Science, 73: 1241-1248.

FAO, (2000). Food safety and quality as affected by animal feedstuff. Twenty second FAO regional conference for Europe, Porto, Portugal, FAO, Rome. pp.4-5.

Galvano, F., Ritieni, A., Piva, G. and Pietri, A. (2005). Mycotoxins in the human food chain *in:* The Mycotoxin Bluebook, *ed.* D. Diaz, Nottingham University Press, Nottingham, UK, pp.187-224

Garaleviciene, D., Pettersson, H., Augonyte, G., Elwinger, K. and Lindberg, J. E. (2001). Effects of mould and toxin contaminated barley on laying hens performance and health. Archives of Animal Nutrition, 55: 25-42.

Garon, D., Richard, E., Sage, L., Bouchart, V., Pottier, D. and Lebailly, P. (2006). Mycoflora and multimycotoxin detection in corn silage: experimental study. Journal of Agricultural and Food Chemistry, 54: 3479-3484.

Gautier, J-C., Holzhaeuser, D., Markovic, J., Grtemaud, E., Schilter, B. and Turesky, R. J. (2001). Oxidative damage and stress response from ochratoxin A exposure in rats. Free Radical Biology and Medicine, 30: 1089-1098.

Gupta, S., Jindal, N., Khokar, R. S., Gupta, A. K., Ledoux, D. R. and Rottinghaus, G. E. (2005). Effect of ochratoxin A on broiler chicks challenged with *Salmonella gallinarum*. British Poultry Science, 46: 443-450.

Hoehler, D., Marquardt, R. R. and Frohlich, A. A. (1997). Lipid peroxidation as one mode of action in ochratoxin A toxicity in rats and chicks. Canadian Journal of Animal Science, 77: 287-292.

Holmberg, T., Kaspersson, A., Larsson, K., and Pettersson, H. (1989). Aflatoxin production in moist barley treated with suboptimal doses of formic and propionic acid. Acta Agricultura. Scandinavica, 39, 457-464.

Hwang, J-H. and Lee, K.-G. (2006). Reduction of aflatoxin B_1 contamination in wheat by various cooking treatments. Food

Chemistry, 98: 71-75.

Jansen van Rensburg, C., Van Rensburg, C. E. J., Van Ryssen, J. B. J., Casey, N. H. and Rottinghaus, G. E. (2006). In vitro and in vivo assessment of humic acid as an aflatoxin binder in broiler chickens. Poultry Science, 85: 1576-1583.

Klein, P. J., Van Vleet, T. R., Hall J. O. and Coulombe Jr., R. A. (2002). Effects of dietary butylated hydroxytoluene on aflatoxin B_1 –relevant metabolic enzymes in turkeys. Food and Chemical Toxicology, 41: 761-678.

Kubena, L. F., Harvey, R. B., Huff, W. E., Corrier, D. E., Phillips, T. D. and Rottinghaus, G. E. (1989). Influence of ochratoxin A and T-2 toxin singly and in combination on broiler chickens. Poultry Science, 68: 867–872.

Kubena, L. F., Edrington, T. S., Harvey, R. B., Phillips, T. D., Sarr, A. B. and Rottinghaus, G. E. (1997). Individual and combined effects of fumonisin B1 present in Fusarium moniliforme culture material and diacetoxyscirpenol or ochratoxin A in turkey poults. Poultry Science, 76: 256–264.

Kumar, A., Jindal, N., Shukla, C. L., Yash Pal, Ledoux, D. R. and Rottinghaus, G. E. (2003). Effect of Ochratoxin A on *Escherichia coli*-challenged broiler chicks. Avian Diseases, 47: 415-424.

Li, Y. C., Ledoux, D. R., Bermudez, A. J., Fritsche, K. L. and Rottinghaus, G. E. (2000a). Effects of moniliformin on performance and immune function of broiler chicks. Poultry Science, 79: 26-32.

Li, Y.C., Ledoux, D. R., Bermudez, A. J., Fritsche, K. L. and Rottinghaus G. E. (2000b). The individual and combined effects of fumonisin B_1 and moniliformin on performance and selected immune parameters in turkey poults. Poultry Science, 79: 871-878.

Lowry, V. K., Farnell, M. B., Ferro, P. J., Swaggerty, C. L., Bahl, A. and Kogut, M. H. (2005). Purified ß-glucan as an abiotic feed additive up-regulates the innate immune response in immature chickens against *Salmonella enterica* serovar *Enteritidis*. International Journal of Food Microbiology, 98: 309-318.

Monroe, D. H., Holeski, C. J. and Eaton, D. L. (1986). Effects of single-dose and repeated-dose treatment with 2(3)-ter-butyl-hydroxyanisole (BHA) on the hepatobiliary disposition and covalent binding to DNA of aflatoxin B_1 in the rat. Food and Chemical Toxicology, 24: 1273-1281.

Nahm, K. H. (1990). Conditions for mould growth and aflatoxin production in feedstuffs. Pig News and Information, 11: 349-352.

Rahnema, S. and Neal, S. M. (1994). Laboratory and field evaluation of commercial feed preservatives in the diet of nursery pigs. Journal of Animal Science. 72: 572-576.

Ramos, A. J. and Hernandéz, E. (1997). Prevention of aflatoxicosis in farm animals by means of hydrated sodium calcium aluminosilicate addition to feedstuffs: a review. Animal Feed Science and Technology, 65: 197-206.

Rizzo, A. F., Atroshi, F., Ahotupa, M., Sankari, S. and Elovaara, E. (1994). Protective effect of antioxidants against free radical-mediated lipid peroxidation induced by DON or T-2 toxin. Journal of Veterinary Medicine A, 41: 81-90.

Schell, T. C., Lindemann, M. D., Kornegay, E. T., Blodgett, D. J. and Doerr, J. A. (1993). Effectiveness of different types of clay for reducing the detrimental effects of aflatoxin-contaminated diets on performance and serum profiles of weanling pigs. Journal of Animal Science, 71: 1226-1231.

Swamy, H. V. L. N. and Devegowda, G. (1998). Ability of mycosorb to counteract aflatoxicosis in commercial broilers. Indian Journal of Poultry Science, 33: 273-278.

Swamy, H. V. L. N., Smith, T. K., MacDonald, E. J., Boermans, H. J. and Squires, E. J. (2002). Effects of feeding a blend of grains naturally contaminated with Fusarium mycotoxins on swine performance, brain regional neurochemistry, and serum chemistry and the efficacy of a polymeric glucomannan mycotoxin adsorbent. Journal of Animal Science, 80: 3257-3267.

Trenholm, H. L., Foster, B. C., Charmley, L. L., Thompson, B. K., Hartin, K. E., Coppock, R. W. and Albassam, M. A. (1994). Effects of feeding diets containing *Fusarium* (naturally) contaminated wheat or pure deoxynivalenol (DON) in growing pigs. Canadian Journal of Animal Science, 74: 361-369.

Valdivia, A. G., Martinez, A., Damián, F. J., Quezada, T., Ortiz, R., Martinez, C., Llamas, J., Rodriguez, M. L., Yamamoto, L., Jaramillo, F., Loarca-Pina, M. G. and Reyes, J. L. (2001). Efficacy of N-acetylcysteine to reduce the effects of aflatoxin B_1 intoxication in broiler chickens. Poultry Science, 80: 727-743.

Yegani, M., Smith, T. K., Leeson, S. and Boermans, H. J. (2006). Effects of feeding grains naturally contaminated with *Fusarium* mycotoxins on performance and metabolism of broiler breeders. Poultry Science, 85: 1541-1549.

5 Feed-Host Interactions (1): Gastrointestinal Integrity

A common characteristic of all living animals is the necessity for the regular consumption of feed which as discussed in Chapter 1, is an extremely complex material. Feed inevitably contains mainly thousands of different molecules and an enormous array of associated micro-organisms. Therefore it is hardly surprising that the nature of feed will have important interactions with the consuming host which in turn will influence Nutrition-based Health (NbH). Feed can interact with the host in at least three different ways and each will be discussed in the next three chapters.

(1) Maintenance of gastrointestinal integrity
(2) Support of the immune system
(3) Modulation of oxidative stress and disease

The gastrointestinal tract is probably the most important organ in an animal. It is an interface with the environment. Feed components in the lumen of the gastrointestinal tract are still outside the body but they exert effects upon animal health and growth and this has been described as External Nutrition (Chapter 1). It is only when nutrients and nutricines are absorbed across the wall of the gastrointestinal tract that they are physiologically inside the body, (Internal Nutrition).

The frequent presence of pathogenic bacteria such as *Escherichia coli, Clostridia perfringens, Lawsonia intracellularis* and viruses, and their proliferation and metabolic activities, will perturb the normal digestive functions of the gastrointestinal tract. This will lead to the onset of various enteric diseases usually characterised by diarrhoea or scouring, poor growth rates and increased mortalities, especially in young animals.

Therefore the development of a complex stable gastrointestinal microflora is important for health maintenance and disease avoidance in animals. It also has a major influence upon performance and productivity of animals raised for food. Establishing optimal conditions in the gastrointestinal ecosystem during stressful periods such as weaning in mammals and hatching and early growth in avian species is of the utmost importance to prevent various enteric disorders.

In the recent past gastrointestinal health of animals raised for food was traditionally managed by various antibiotics and other drugs. However the final prohibition of antibiotic growth promoters in the EU in 2006 together with the high profile of food safety amongst consumers have required changes in strategies to maintain good gastrointestinal health.

Therefore it is very important to develop nutritional strategies which maintains and supports gastrointestinal integrity.

The gastrointestinal tract has five major functions as shown in Table 1.

Table 1. The functions of the gastrointestinal tract.

Function	*Description*
Defence barrier	The wall of the gastrointestinal tract is the ultimate barrier between the external environment and the internal body tissues.
Colonization resistance	Establishment of a stable microflora which can inhibit the growth of invading pathogenic micro-organisms.
Digestion	Physical and enzymatic breakdown of large molecular weight feed materials into small nutrient units such as sugars, amino acids and fatty acids. .
Absorption	Transfer of digested nutrients into the tissues of the body.
Fermentation	Primarily in the large intestine
Elimination	Removal of undigested dietary components.

Defence barrier

The cells of the gastrointestinal tract are the last line in the body's defence against pathogenic organisms and toxins arriving in feed or water. Feed ingredients, as well as toxins and micro-organisms frequently have the potential to damage the structure of the gastrointestinal tract. This leads to various enteric disease problems such as coccidiosis, necrotic enteritis and poult enteritis and mortality syndrome as discussed in Chapter 3. Collectively these are manifested as malabsorption of nutrients, diarrhoea and wet litter, poor growth and performance and sometimes increased mortalities.

In chicks the development of the gastrointestinal tract is associated with the beginning of feeding. After five days growth chicks which were given feed and water immediately had a significantly greater small intestine mass of 10.6 g compared to a small intestine mass of only 8.68g in those chicks denied feed and water for the first 24 hours (Mikec *et al.,* 2006).

The functional development of the gastrointestinal tract is also related to its development as a major site of the immune system, the gut associated lymphoid tissue (GALT). The GALT provides protection against pathogens arriving in the gastrointestinal tract. Development of the GALT was delayed in the large intestine in chicks suffering from feed deprivation (Shira *et al.*, 2005). Full development of the GALT occurred by two weeks of age but this also means that for a two week period chicks with delayed access to feed would be more vulnerable to environmental pathogens those fed immediately. For optimum chick growth and development feed and water must be offered without any delay immediately upon arrival at the farms.

Although maintenance of the health of the gastrointestinal tract is extremely important, it is also very complex. It relies on a delicate balance between the mucosa, which includes the digestive epithelium, GALT and the overlying mucus layer, the intestinal microflora and the diet. These components interact with each other to form a delicate and dynamic equilibrium within the gastrointestinal tract that ensures efficient functioning of the digestive system. In addition a number of protective proteins such as immunoglobulin A, various growth factors and cytokines interact with the mucus layer at the mucosal surface.

The internal structure of the wall of the gastrointestinal tract and in particular the mucus layer are important in maintaining an effective protective barrier function. The entire luminal surface of the gastrointestinal tract is covered with a mucus layer which is mainly composed of a large molecular weight glycoprotein, mucin. It is particularly rich in the amino acids threonine, serine and proline with a carbohydrate fraction based on galactose, fucose, N-acetlyglucosamine, N-acetylgalactosamine and sialic acid (Lien *et al.*, 2001)(Table 2). The large amount of carbohydrate residues in mucus probably make it resistant to proteolytic digestion.

Table 2. The composition of gastric and small intestinal mucins from pigs.

Component	*Mucin orign*	
	Stomach (gastric)	*Small intestine*
General composition (%DM)		
Carbohydrate	78.0	54.1
Protein	15.4	21.2
Sialic acid	2.9	21.6
Sulphate	3.7	3.1
Protein composition (mol/100mol)		
Proline	16.0	16.4
Serine	18.1	12.1
Threonine	18.3	27.2
Carboydrate composition (mol/100mol)		
Fucose	17.4	9.6
Galactose	39.9	26.5
N-acetylglucosamine	29.9	22.6
N-acetylgalactosamine	12.8	41.3

In healthy animals the mucus layer is in a dynamic balance. Loss of mucus from the gastrointestinal lumen wall is compensated by synthesis and secretion of mucins from specialized differentiated cells known as goblet cells distributed throughout the epithelium (Montagne, *et al.*, 2004). Mucins found in the digesta in the lumen of the gastrointestinal tract are a result of either proteolytic digestion or abrasion of the mucus layer. In the lumen however the mucin is partially protected from further proteolysis by the oligosaccharide component that covers much of the protein backbone of the mucin. This mucin is therefore poorly digested in the small intestine and could represent an important proportion of the endogenous protein that reaches the large intestine and is thereby lost to the animal.

Mucus together with bicarbonate protects the epithelium of the gastrointestinal tract from vigorous digestive processes and corrosive gastric juices by creating an unstirred layer and acting as a diffusion barrier, preventing large molecular weight compounds such as proteolytic enzymes from reaching the epithelium. Mucus traps toxins and bacteria preventing infection. It also plays an important role in the digestive processes by creating a digestive zone in which enzymes are immobilized near the epithelial surface, preventing their rapid removal by peristalsis and placing them in a more favourable position for digestion (Lien *et al.*, 2001).

Feed consumption increases mucus synthesis and conversely feed restriction reduces it. Reducing feed intake in rats to half the normal daily intake resulted in a dramatic decrease in mucus production (Sherman *et al.*, 1985). Mucin isolated from malnourished rats was chemically similar to that found in control animals. Therefore malnutrition resulted in an absolute decrease in intestinal mucin rather than in any molecular changes. It is likely that this impaired mucin production induced by malnutrition would also be an important factor in reducing intestinal resistance to enteric diseases.

Reduced feed intake as often seen in post-weaning piglets may well lead to reduced mucus production which may increase their susceptibilmity to enteric diseases. Dietary fibre also has an impact upon mucus production with a greater secretion of mucus in animals fed diets containing insoluble rather than soluble fibre. Adequate feed intake with some insoluble fibre will be important to maintain good levels of mucus synthesis. This in turn should lead to good intestinal health.

Mucins are substantial constituents of the basal endogenous protein in the gastrointestinal tract. Dietary strategies that increase mucin synthesis might be beneficial to protect against pathogens and will be important to protect and to maintain the functional integrity of the gastrointestinal tract. However increased mucin synthesis would also increase the maintenance requirement for amino acids, particularly threonine, and for energy. This would decrease the availability of these nutrients for animal growth and production. More work is needed to demonstrate that manipulating mucin through feeding strategies would enhance animal health. It would be an attractive part of an NbH strategy.

Microflora and colonization resistance

Interactions between the mucus layer and bacteria in the gastrointestinal tract are very important in terms of animal health. Many commensal and pathogenic bacteria adhere to complex carbohydrates in the mucus layer. The binding of commensal bacteria prevents colonization by opportunistic pathogens. This is the colonization resistance effect of the mucus layer.

The diet of an animal is an important factor controlling the composition and metabolic activities of the microflora in the gastrointestinal tract (Bauer *et al.*, 2006). Fermentable carbohydrates seem to be most promising in terms of promoting the proliferation of beneficial bacterial species. Carbohydrate fermentation yields short chain fatty acids which have health-promoting effects. Fermentation of proteins on the other hand, is often associated with growth of potential pathogens, and results in the production of detrimental substances including ammonia and amines. Various medium chain fatty acids also have antimicrobial activities. The intestinal microflora can be divided into three groups:

Commensal ⟷ Symbiotic ⟷ Pathogenic

The individual bacterial species in these groups are not irrevocably fixed and some commensal bacteria may at times become pathogenic or symbiotic. The final microbiological flora of the gastrointestinal tract reflects the co-evolution of micro-organisms with the animal host and the feed consumed by the host. Most pathogens need to arrive in large numbers or to grow rapidly to overcome the resident microflora's resistance to colonization. However, if the stable microflora is disrupted there is an increased risk of infection, either by an invading pathogen or by a normal resident of the gastrointestinal tract, which has previously been maintained at low numbers by the interactions between various species in the gastrointestinal tract.

There is an enormous diversity of the micoflora in the gastrointestinal tract as illustrated by the isolation of 1,230 partial 16S rRNA gene sequences from the gastrointestinal tract of broilers, (Lu *et al.*, 2003). In the ileum, there were predominantly four groups comprising *Lactobacilli* 70%, *Clostridiaceae*, 11%, *Streptococcus*, 6.6% and *Enterococcus*, 6.5%. In the caecum, *Clostidiaceae* were the most abundant group comprising 65% of the total. This large predominance of clostridial species was previously relatively unknown.

The microflora in the gastrointestinal tract makes an important contribution to overall animal health. It provides a continuous stimulus to the gut associated lymphoid tissues which comprise the immune system in the gastrointestinal tract. The commensal microflora also restricts the establishment of pathogenic bacteria which have to compete with the indigenous microflora for nutrition and binding sites.

Fermentation in the large intestine

Fermentation is well recognised as an important aspect of nutrient utilization in ruminants. However, it is also important in the caecum and the colon of monogastric animals which comprises the large intestine. The functions of the large intestine were considered for many years to be primarily the conservation of water and electrolytes. However it is now appreciated that an important activity is the salvage of energy and nutrients through the fermentative activities of the microflora inhabiting the large intestine. Although digestion by endogenous enzymes and absorption of nutrients from the small intestine is very efficient there is still a constant supply of nutrients to the large intestine in the form of undigested dietary components, host enzymes, mucus fragments and intestinal mucosal cells.

The amount and composition of substances reaching the large intestine can be readily modified by diet (Williams, *et al.,* 2001). The fermentable carbohydrate fraction of the feed such as non-digestible oligosaccharide, non-starch polysaccharides and resistant starch are the most important bacterial substrates. The end products of fermentation are the volatile fatty acids (VFA); acetic, propionic and butyric which are readily absorbed from the large intestine together with the non-volatile fatty acid, lactic acid, which tends to be poorly absorbed from the large intestine. The VFA are valuable nutrients for the enterocytes in the large intestine with butyric acid being the most important. Butyric acid is also required for the normal development of epithelial cells (Pryde *et al.*, 2002). Sodium butyrate increases the mucin synthesis of colon tissue, *in vitro,* with a maximum effect at a concentration of 0.1 mM (Finnie *et al.*, 1995). This very significant increase in mucin synthesis from addition of sodium butyrate to a standard nutrient medium, suggests that that this may be an important mechanisms affecting the rate of mucin synthesis and may also explain the therapeutic effect of butyrate in colitis. Butyrate also has a potent anti-inflammatory effect both *in vivo* and *in vitro* (Andoh *et al.,* 1999). Butyric acid and its salts are currently used in some feed formulations, although the unpleasant odour of butyric acid limits its application in many animal feeds.

The VFA and lactic acid have potent antibacterial activities, particularly against Gram negative pathogens such as *E. coli* and *Salmonella* spp. Consequently there may well be advantages in gastrointestinal health through the maintenance of a good basal level of the VFA and lactic acid in the large intestine.

If the carbohydrate sources in the large intestine become depleted the fermentation becomes more and more proteolytic. This can lead to the formation of potentially toxic metabolites such as ammonia, amines, volatile phenols and indoles which occur only in small amounts in the healthy large intestine.

The micoflora in the large intestine contribute significantly to the utilization of nutrients which escape digestion and absorption in the small intestine.

Amino acids

Several amino acids; arginine, glutamine, histidine, and threonine are known to play an important role in maintaining the integrity of the gastrointestinal tract. Most animal feeds are formulated to include specific amounts only of lysine and methionine and in some cases threonine is considered. However the amino acid content of feeds is usually only considered from the growth point of view rather from an NbH approach.

Arginine plays an important role in tissue repair and immune cell function (Corzo *et al.,* 2003). It is also a substrate for nitric oxide (NO) synthase in macrophages which is an important part of the innate immune system. Unfortunately the high cost of arginine limits its application in animal feeds

Glutamine is the most abundant amino acid found in mammalian blood and in the free amino acid pool of the body. It plays an important role in inter-organ nitrogen transport, as a nitrogen donor for the synthesis of nucleotides and amino-sugars. It is a key substrate for renal ammonia formation. Glutamine is a major metabolic fuel for the mucosa in the gastrointestinal tract by generating ATP through oxidation. In times of severe disease or inflammation, glutamine frequently becomes a conditionally essential amino acid because utilization may exceed synthesis.

Glutamine is important in maintaining the gastrointestinal mucosa and it prevented damage to the villi during the first week post weaning in piglets (GuoYao *et al.,* 1996). In mice with gut-derived sepsis dietary glutamine supplementation enhanced lymphocyte function and reduced myeloperoxidase activity in several organs. This indicated that glutamine was able to reduce the extent of tissue injury in mice with sepsis. Weaning piglets fed a glutamine supplemented diet showed an improved barrier function in the gastrointestinal tract and better mucosal repair (Domeneghini *et al.*, 2006). There is considerable evidence that dietary glutamine is very beneficial in maintaining integrity of the gastrointestinal tract.

Histidine inhibited the secretion of inflammatory cytokines in gastrointestinal cells suffering from an oxidative stress (Son *et al.*, 2005). This oxidative stress leads to the onset of a range of inflammatory diseases which will disturb the normal functioning of the gastrointestinal tract. In this experiment histidine was much more effective than other amino acids such as lysine, proline, glutamine, alanine and γ-aminobutyric acid. Histidine could therefore be an important anti-inflammatory agent in the gastrointestinal tract and help to maintain normal, stable conditions.

Threonine is strongly associated with metabolism of the gastrointestinal tract. An adequate level of dietary threonine is crucial for mucin production and maintenance of the integrity of the gastrointestinal function in piglets (Le Floc'h *et al.* 2004).

Enteric health in poultry: malabsorption syndrome (MAS)

A single causative agent for MAS has not yet been found and it is recognized as being a multifactorial disease involving a combination of pathogens. These may be various viruses such as reovirus, adenovirus, rotavirus and parvovirus together with bacteria such as *Escherichia coli, Proteus mirabilis, Enterococcus faecium* and *Clostridia perfringens* (Rebel *et al.*, 2006). However none of these agents are capable of causing the disease by itself.

It is quite an economically important disease in broiler production and has a worldwide occurrence. Infected birds have a decreased body weight gain, increased mortality, downgraded carcass quality and are frequently susceptible to secondary diseases. Flocks suffering from MAS have widespread stunting and uneven growth. There is frequently diarrhea with excretion of undigested feed resulting in wet litter, retarded feathering, pigment loss and bone abnormalities.

The MAS has been given a variety of other names such as infectious proventriculitis, runting and stunting syndrome or pale bird syndrome. Birds suffering from MAS have a reduced ability to absorb dietary carotenoids. They will have pale shanks, hence the term "pale bird syndrome," and will have an excessive excretion of carotenoids in the faeces. This will have serious economic consequences in the production of pigmented or yellow broilers.

Although the disease is known as MAS it is not in fact clearly established whether it is a problem of impaired feed digestion, impaired absorption of digested nutrients, or both. Factors that influence the induction and severity of MAS are the genetic background of the broiler, the health status of the one-day old chicks, nutrition, environmental stress and management. (Rebel *et al.*, 2004).

Birds infected with MAS develop severe enteritis. This is associated with impaired enzymatic digestion and the development of lesions in the small intestine. It has also been noted that the greatest susceptibility to MAS is the first two weeks of age. This is the same period in which there is rapid development of the enterocytes in the gastrointestinal tract and the systemic immune system is not fully developed. Differences in the development of the innate and adaptive immunity at an early age could be a crucial factor in the onset of MAS.

The modern broiler has been extensively selected for fast body weight gain. However there may also have been other indirect selections made which may result in a decrease in general resistance leading to disease susceptibility or an adverse adaptation against enteric disorders (Chapter 1). The onset of MAS is probably related to an immune response such as the production of inflammatory cytokines and the influx of heterophils into mucosal tissue in the gastrointestinal tract.

Enteric health in pigs

Health maintenance and disease avoidance in animals requires a stable and resilient microflora in the gastrointestinal tract. Therefore it is important to avoid abrupt changes in diet that may destabilise the microflora in the gastrointestinal tract (Hillman, 2004). However in modern pig production there is an inevitable disruption to the microflora and to the structure of the gastrointestinal tract at weaning. In piglets weaning is associated with an abrupt change from milk to solid food. The casein and lactose in milk are suddenly replaced by plant proteins and starch, which destabilises the gastrointestinal microflora and makes the animals susceptible to various enteric disorders.

Enteric diseases of weaning piglets remains a major animal health problem and is constantly under active research. Various dietary manipulations to control or avoid enteric disorders in weaning piglets has already been presented in Chapter 3. A possible strategy to maintain piglet health is to incorporate significant quantities of lactose or the non-digestible oligosaccharide, inulin into the diet (Pierce *et al.*, 2006). A diet containing 33% lactose compared to 15%, showed increased volatile fatty acid production in the caecum and an increased population of *Lactobacilli* with a slight reduction in *E. coli* (Table 3). These are positive health benefits. The inclusion of 15% inulin with 15% lactose also showed beneficial health effects in terms of reduced intestinal pH and increase in villous height. A combination of high lactose and inulin however resulted in a reduction in faecal dry matter, lactobacilli and bifidobacteria concentrations. This was probably due to an excessive quantity of carbohydrate entering the colon that exceeded the fermentative capacity of the piglet.

Table 3. The effect of increased dietary lactose on total volatile fatty acids (VFA) in digesta water concentration and on the populations of *Lactobacilli* and *E. coli* in the caecum and colon of weanling pigs.

Location	*Parameter*	*Dietary lactose (%)*	
		15	*33*
Caecum	Total VFA mmol/l)	94.8	163.2
	Lactobacilli (log_{10} colony forming units/g)	6.3	7.2
	E. coli (log_{10} colony forming units/g)	7.1	6.3
Colon	Total VFA mmol/l)	99.9	194.2
	Lactobacilli (log_{10} colony forming units/g)	6.4	7.4
	Lactobacilli (log_{10} colony forming units/g)	7.2	6.5

Lactoferrin, a multifunctional glycoprotein obtained from milk, gave beneficial effects on the gastrointestinal morphology of weaned piglets (Wang *et al.*, 2006). When lactoferrin was incorporated into piglet feeds at 1 kg/tonne there was a greater villus height and reduced crypt depth in the small intestine indicative of improved health of the gastrointestinal tract. Lactoferrin has many physiological roles including protection against microbial infection and regulation of immune function and might well offer useful benefits in piglet nutrition.

Conclusions

The gastrointestinal tract is a major organ in the body and forms an interface with the external environment. The integrity of the gastrointestinal tract is a major health determinant as enteric diseases cause serious problems and economic losses in animal production. Development of the gastrointestinal tract is related to the supply of feed and delay in feeding of poultry can affect normal growth and development. The internal luminal surface of the gastrointestinal tract is covered with a mucus layer. This protects the epithelium from damage through digestive processes or toxins in the feed. Adequate feed intake is important to maintain the integrity of the mucus layer. There is a very extensive microflora which develops in the gastrointestinal tract and this contributes to protection against pathogens and also to fermentation of undigested feed components in the large intestine. Fermentation products, particularly butyric acid, are valuable nutrients for the enterocytes in the large intestine. Several amino acids such as arginine, glutamine, threonine and histidine help to maintain the integrity of the gastrointestinal tract. Enteric diseases such as malabsorption syndrome in broilers and various scouring problems in piglets are manifestations of disturbances in the gastrointestinal tract.

References

Andoh, A., Bamba, T., and Sasaki, M. (1999). Physiological and anti-inflammatory roles of dietary fibre and butyrate in intestinal functions. Journal of Parenteral and Enteral Nutrition, 23: S70-S73.

Bauer, E., Williams, B. A., Smidt, H., Mosenthin, R. and Verstegen, M. W. A. (2006). Influence of dietary components on development of the microbiota in single-stomached species. Nutrition Research Reviews, 19: 63-78.

Corzo, A., Moran, E. T. and Hoehler, D. (2003). Arginine need of heavy broiler males: Applying the ideal protein concept. Poultry Science, 82: 402-407.

Domeneghini, C., Giancillo, A. di, and Bosi, G. (2006). Can nutraceuticals affect the structure of intestinal mucosa? Qualitative and quantitative microanatomy in L-glutamine diet-supplemented weaning piglets. Veterinary Research Communications, 30: 331-342.

Finnie, I. A., Dwarakanath, A. D., Taylor, B. A. and Rhodes, J. M. (1995). Colonic mucin synthesis is increased by sodium butyrate. Gut, 36: 93-99.

GuoYao, W., Meier, S. A. and Knabe, D. A. (1996). Dietary glutamine supplementation prevents atrophy in weaned piglets. Journal of Nutrition, 126: 2578-2584.

Hillman, K. (2004). Effect of raw materials on bacterial control of the gut. *In* Disease Control Without Medicines, Society of Feed Technologists, UK.

Le Floc'h, N., Melchior, D. and Obled, C. (2004). Modification of protein and amino acid metabolism during inflammation and immune system activation. Livestock Production Science, 87: 37-45.

Lien, K. A., Sauer, W. C. and He, J. M. (2001). Dietary influences on the secretion into and degradation of mucin in the digestive tract of monogastric animals and humans. Journal of Animal and Feed Sciences, 10: 223-245.

Lu, J., Idris, U., Harmon, B., Hofacre, C., Maurer, J. L. and Lee, M. D. (2003). Diversity and succession of the intestinal bacterial community of the maturing broiler chicken. Applied and Environmental Microbiology, 69: 6816-6824.

Mikec, M., Bidin, Z., Valentic´, A., Savic´ V., Zelenika, A. T., Raguz-Duric´, R. Novak, I. L. and Balenovic M. (2006). Influence of environment and nutritional stressors on yolk sac utilization, development of chicken gastrointestinal system and its immune status. World's Poultry Science Journal, 62: 31-40.

Montagne, L., Piel, C. and Lallès, J. P. (2004). Effect of diet on mucin kinetics and composition: nutrition and health implications. Nutrition

Reviews, 62: 105-114.

Pierce, K. M., Sweeney, T., Brophy, P. O., Callan, J. J., Fitzpatrick, E., McCarthy, P and O'Doherty, J. V. (2006). The effect of lactose and inulin on intestinal morphology, selected microbial populations and volatile fatty acid concentrations in the gastro-intestinal tract of the weanling pig. Animal Science, 82:311-318.

Pryde, S. E., Duncan, S. H., Hold, G. L., Stewart, C. S. and Flint, H. J. (2002). The microbiology of butyrate formation in the human colon. FEMS Microbiology Letters, 217: 133-139.

Rebel, J. M. J., van Dam, J. T. P., Zekarias, B., Balk, F. R. M., Post, J., Flores minambres, A. and ter Huurne, A. A. H. M. (2004). Vitamin and trace mineral content in feed of breeders and their progeny: effects of growth, feed conversion and severity of malabsorption syndrome of broilers. British Poultry Science, 45: 201-209.

Rebel, J. M. J., Balk, F. R. M., Post, J., Van Hemert, S., Zekarias, B and Stockhofe, N. (2006). Malabsorption syndrome in broilers. World's Poultry Science Journal, 62 : 17-29.

Sherman, P., Forstner, J., Roomi, N., Khatri, I. And Forstner, G. (1985). Mucin depletion in the intestine of malnourished rats. American Journal of Physiology-Gastrointestinal and Liver Physiology, 248: G418-423.

Shira, E. B., Sklan, D. and Friedman, A. (2005). Impaired immune response in broiler hatchling hindgut following delayed access to feed. Veterinary Immunology and Immunopathology, 105: 33-35.

Son, D. O., Satsu, H. and Shimizu, M. (2005). Histidine inhibits oxidative stress- and TNF-a-induced inteleukin-8 secretion in intestinal epithelial cells. FEBS Letters, 579: 4671-4677.

Wang, Y., Shan, T., Xu, Z., Liu, J. and Feng, J. (2006). Effect of lactoferrin on the growth performance, intestinal morphology and expression of PR-39 and protegrin-1 genes in weaned piglets. Journal of Animal Science, 84: 2636-2641.

Williams, B. A., Verstegen, M. W. A. and Tamminga, S. (2001). Fermentation in the large intestine of single-stomached animals and its relationship to animal health. Nutrition Research Reviews, 14: 207-227.

6 Feed-Host Interactions (2): Support the Immune System

Animals inevitably live in a hostile environment and they are exposed to an enormous range of micro-organisms, which occur in feed, water and the environment. Some pathogenic micro-organisms readily penetrate the epithelia of the respiratory, gastrointestinal and genital systems and invade the body. Many micro-organisms live in the gastrointestinal tract and other cavities of most animals. The huge bacterial population in the gastrointestinal tract can be beneficial or deleterious to the health of the animal and must be well-managed. Virus infections of the gastrointestinal tract occur commonly in pigs and poultry and can cause little or no symptoms, or they can lead to catastrophic losses. Furthermore virus infections of the gastrointestinal tract are likely to encourage the development of other diseases. Viruses may damage the mucosal lining of the gastrointestinal tract and provide an access point for other potential pathogens such as *E. Coli* or *Salmonella* spp. Such damage may also allow attachment of other pathogens to the wall of the gastrointestinal tract. Damage to the gastrointestinal tract and the onset of diarrhoea syndromes caused by various pathogens will also have a secondary effect upon the ability of the infected animal to digest and absorb nutrients.

Growth of pathogenic micro-organisms must be controlled to avoid direct disease syndromes, opportunistic infections and severe enteric disorders. Therefore a second important feed-host interaction is the influence of diet in supporting the immune system.

(1) Maintenance of gastrointestinal integrity
(2) Support the immune system
(3) Modulation of oxidative stress and disease

The policy of eradication of animal diseases through hygiene and slaughter strategies brings an associated risk that that livestock become naïve to certain pathogens and as a consequence become susceptible to epidemic outbreaks. Also there is an increasing tendency in many countries to reduce the use of antibiotics and other drugs in animal production to control infectious diseases. Consequently the development and support of an efficient immune system becomes increasingly important to protect animal health.

Infection by pathogenic micro-organisms impacts very closely upon nutrition as illustrated in Figure 1. Suppression of appetite reduces nutrient intake which is of major importance in maintenance of good animal growth. Damage to the tissues of the gastrointestinal tract may occur, either to the villi as frequently occurs in weaning piglets or possibly through development of lesions such as in necrotic enteritis in poultry. Theses damages are manifested as diarrhoea and malabsorption of nutrients from the feed. The overall result is a loss of ingested nutrients which should be used for growth. Increased body temperature and activation of the immune system increases the nutrient requirement, but these nutrients are not used to support growth of the animal body.

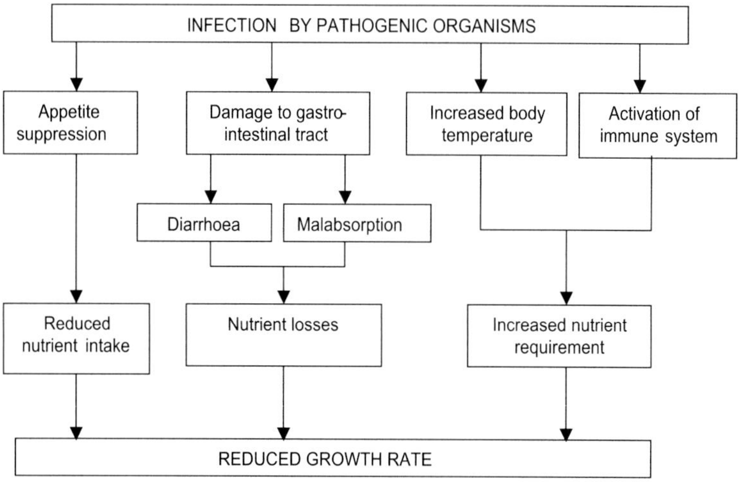

Figure 1. Effects of infection by pathogenic organisms which result in reduced growth rates of animals.

A compromised immunity in animals raised for food will obviously result in reduced production efficiency through increased susceptibility to diseases, morbidity and mortality. However the immune response also has to be tightly controlled otherwise serious inflammatory disease could develop and also the immune response is growth inhibiting. Therefore immunomodulation measures in food animals will remain extremely important in maintenance of animal health. In particular there will be more emphasis on mucosal immunity and the activation of the innate immune system through nutritional strategies

The innate immune response is critical to enteric disease resistance and to the induction of mucosal adaptive immunity. This arm of the immune system consists of natural killer (NK) cells, granulocytes, macrophages and mast cells. It provides an important front line of protection against microbial pathogens since it is a very rapid defence mechanism and NK cells in particular are important for the protection against viruses.

The activation of the innate immune system depends upon the recognition of specific microbial signature molecules called pathogen-associated molecular patterns (PAMPs). These PAMPs are not found in the host cells but occur in many micro-organisms. These include molecules such as lipopolysaccharide, bacterial lipopeptides, double-stranded RNA, and DNA bearing unmethylated CpG motifs.

Among the mediators of the innate immune system which recognise these PAMPs are the Toll-like receptors (TLRs) (Takeda *et al.*, 2003). The response of cells of the gastrointestinal tract to microbial PAMPs, depends upon the expression of TLRs on the cell surface. This results in the activation of macrophages which produce reactive oxygen and nitrogen species that have an antimicrobial effect. There is also an activation of transcription factors, mainly nuclear factor kappa B (NF-κB), through adaptor molecules and downstream kinases such as IRAK-4. This system controls the production of proinflamatory cytokines which stimulates the adaptive immune response. The innate immune system response will either inhibit the growth and replication of the pathogen or it would initiate a cascade reaction leading to the production of antibodies in the adaptive immune response (Figure 2). This ensures that the host responds in a rapid and appropriate fashion to the microbial challenge.

Figure 2. Schematic of the innate immune system response.

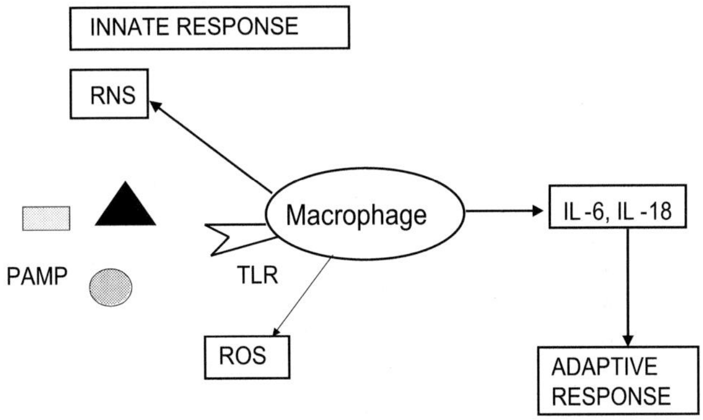

IL: Interleukin,TLR: Toll-like receprtor, PAMP: Pathogen-associated molecular patterns, RNS: Reactive nitrogen species,ROS: Reactive oxygen species

Vertebrates also rely upon the adaptive or the cell mediated immunity where there are two major type of lymphocytes the T-cells and B-cells. Cell-mediated immunity is manifested through the production of antibodies that are released by B-cells into the bloodstream. This immunity is based on the production of immunoglobulins which are able to recognise and eliminate specific antigens such as invading bacteria. This is of necessity much slower than the innate immune system because it requires the production of suitable antibodies to neutralise the pathogens.

The cell-mediated immune system is also responsible for the development of specific immunity as the antibodies produced in response to a pathogen invasion remain in the body for some time and can then protect against a subsequent invasion. Cell-mediated immunity adapts to the pathogen and has memory. The general immune system response is illustrated in Figure 3.

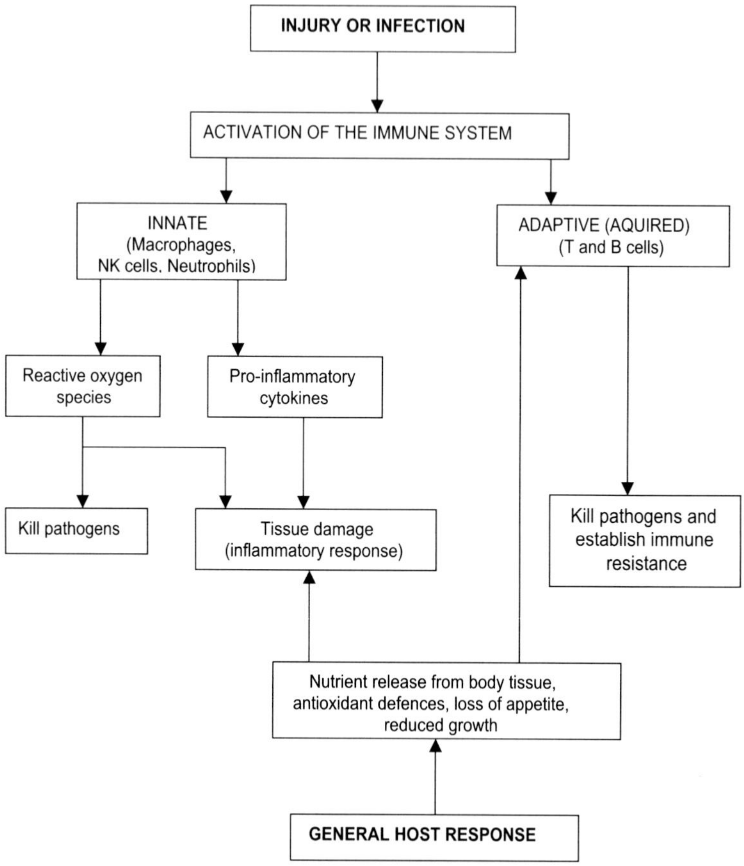

Figure 3. General immune system response.

There is considerable evidence that in both mammalian and in avian species the immune system responds to numerous factors. Some of these are: environment, physiological state, genetic make-up, presence of toxins and nutrition. There is a reciprocal interaction between diet and the immune system, as nutrition modulates the immune system and the immune system responses modulate nutritional needs. Various components in feed such as mycotoxins, bacteria, viruses and nutricines have an important influence upon the immune system. The multisystemic wasting disease (PMWS) of pigs is a condition associated with immune responses and a virus. Mycotoxins as discussed in Chapter 4 are widely recognised as suppressing the immune system (Li *et al.*, 2000a; Li *et al.*, 2000b). Chicks from breeding hens fed aflatoxin showed a serious reduction in immune competetency (Qureshi *et al.*, 1998a). Immunosuppression makes animals more susceptible to secondary infections or to sub-clinical infections and gives poor response to vaccines.

Immunomodulation is an important but delicate aspect of animal production as it requires the avoidance of immunosuppression which would expose the animal to infectious disease, yet it must also avoid excessive activation of the immune system as that is growth-inhibiting. Activation of the immune system may occur during disease challenge or exposure to a high microbial burden in an unhygienic environment. There are several important physiological consequences of this activation of the immune system: production of pro-inflammatory cytokines such as interleukin 1 (IL-1), interleukin 6 (IL-6) and tumour necrosis factor α (TNF-α), development of fever and reduced appetite

It is well accepted that the nature of diet influences the robustness of the immune system but it is still not clear as to how various nutricines and nutrients specifically affect the immune system. Clearly the operation of effective immune responses in an animal requires a supply of nutrients and nutricines at the appropriate times and in the appropriate amounts. However it is not clearly established whether or not the dietary requirements established to maintain growth and reproduction are adequate to support the immune response. It may be that the commonly used nutrient specifications are inadequate for optimal disease resistance since immune system activation and the development of inflammation alter protein metabolism (Le Floc'h *et al.*, 2004).

Low but constant activation of the immune system in animals results in decreased performance since amino acids are diverted away from protein production, which reduces growth and lactation, and towards tissues involved in inflammation and immune response. The dietary amino acids are used for the synthesis of inflammatory and immune proteins, to support immune cell proliferation, and for the synthesis of other compounds important for body defence functions such as acute phase proteins (Chapter 8).

Therefore stimulation of the immune system induces specific requirements for amino acids such as glutamine, cysteine, arginine, tyrosine, phenylalanine and tryptophan and there may well be a benefit from increasing the dietary supply of these amino acids for animals under an immunological stress. Furthermore activation of the immune system is generally associated with a reduced feed intake which would exacerbate any nutritional deficiencies.

Large molecular weight compounds such as polysaccharides, proteins, glycopepetides and nucleotides have been identified as having immunomodulatory properties. Sodium alginate at a dose rate of 2 kg/tonne of shrimp feed enhanced the immune status of white shrimp and increased their resistance to the pathogen *Vibrio alginolyticus* (Cheng *et al.*, 2005). Beta-glucans from yeast cell walls are already used in aquaculture as immunostimulants and have also been shown to up-regulate the innate immunes response in immature chickens against *Salmonella* (Lowry *et al.* 2005). Limited treatment of broiler chickens with a ß-1,3/1,6–glucan from yeast cell wall was able to decrease production losses due to an *Escherichia coli* induced respiratory disease (Huff *et al.,* 2006). However the body weights of non-challenged birds fed the glucan also decreased. This was most likely due to an excessive immune stimulation by the glucans which was growth inhibiting. This is a useful example of the delicacy of immunomodulation. Mushroom and herb polysaccharides incorporated into chicken diets were able to enhance the immune responses in birds infected with the coccidial micro-organism, *Eimeria tenella* (Guo *et al.*, 2004). There was a significantly higher production of specific immunoglobulins; IgA, IgM and IgC in birds infected with *E. tenella* and fed the polysaccharides compared to birds infected with *E. tenella* and not fed the polysaccharides. An oat ß-glucan was able to enhance resistance of immune suppressed mice to infection with *Eimeria verliformis* (Yun *et al.* 1997). Groups of mice were immunosuppressed, infected with *E.vermiformis* and treated with oat ß-glucan. Faecal oocyst shedding was reduced in the ß-glucan-treated groups compared to the control group. Immunosuppressed mice which received no ß-glucan treatment showed more severe clinical signs of coccidiosis disease and a 50% mortality, whilst minimal clinical signs and no mortality were recorded in the ß-glucan-treated groups. This resistance to the *E. vermiformis* organism was also associated with higher levels of a range of immunoglobulins in the blood serum of ß-glucan-treated animals.

Beta-glucans have also been used in pig nutrition with varying results. Improvements in nutrient digestibility and growth performance was not achieved by adding 0.02% ß-glucan to piglet feeds (Hahn *et al.,* 2006). Furthermore there were only marginal benefits seen on the immune parameters of piglets fed ß-glucans. A ß-glucan extracted from yeast, (*Saccharomyces cerevisiae*), gave some improved growth performance at 50 mg/kg feed but higher levels reduced average daily gain (Li *et al.*, 2006). Diets supplemented with 50 mg/kg of ß-glucan partially suppressed increases in concentrations of TNF-a and interleukin-6 and enhanced the increase of interleukin-10 in plasma when the pigs were challenged with lipopolysaccharide. Another source of ß-glucan, from the Chinese herb, *Astragalus membranaceus*, when fed to piglets at 500 g/tonne of feed, decreased the release of the inflammatory cytokines, interleukin-I, prostaglandin E_2 and cortisol (Mao *et al.,* 2005). Such a response would not only decrease the muscle wasting process commonly associated with an immune challenge and the process of nutrient repartitioning from tissue growth to support immune function, but it would also alleviate immune stress. In this example the ß-glucan from *Astragalus membranaceus,* had the potential to improve the immune function of piglets fed in conventional environments.

Various antioxidants, in particular the carotenoids (Chew, 1993; Blount, 2004), and tocopherols are valuable in supporting the immune system. The yellow carotenoid, lutein, modulated cell-mediated and humoral immune responses in cats (Kim *et al.*, 2000a). Feeding cats from 1-10 mg lutein/d gave a significant increase in immunoglobulin G (IgG) production after eight weeks of feeding and this trend persisted up to 12 weeks. Dietary lutein also enhanced antibody response of dogs given routine vaccinations(Kim *et al.*, 2000b).

There is evidence of an immune response to lutein in avian species (Blount *et al.*, 2003). Zebra finches were given a high lutein diet and then challenged with the lectin, phytohaemagglutinin. This lectin induces a cell-mediated immune response which can be measured as a swelling on the skin of the bird. Birds on lutein-supplemented diets showed a two-fold increase in total plasma carotenoids and produced a significantly larger immune response than control birds (Table 1). This suggests that immune function may be limited by carotenoid availability in the diet.

Table 1. Effect of dietary lutein on total plasma carotenoids and an immune response.

Parameter	*Treatment*	
	Control	*Lutein*
Total plasma carotenoids (μg/ml)	32.0	68.0
Immune response (mm)	0.80	1.75

Further support for the implication of lutein in health comes from observations on the inflammatory response in growing chicks (Koutsos *et al.*, 2006). In this study lutein did not influence chick growth *per se* but it blunted indices of systemic inflammatory immune response when chicks were stimulated with lipopolysaccharide (LPS). Chicks that were not fed dietary lutein had greater bodyweight reduction, and greater increases in bursa, thymus and spleen weights post challenge with LPS, than chicks fed lutein. Chicks deficient in lutein had greater acute phase protein response in the blood after the LPS challenge. In laying hens lutein supplementation stimulated an antibody response to infectious bronchitis virus vaccination (Bédécarrats and Leeson, 2006). This suggest that an added benefit of lutein is to increase the efficacy of vaccination. Many poultry feeds, particularly in Europe, will be extremely low in carotenoid content as they are frequently based on wheat, barley and hybrid maize and such diets may not support an optimum immune system.

Supplemental vitamin E when fed to broiler breeders enhanced the lymphocyte function of day old chicks (Haq *et al.*, 1996). There was an increase in antibody production against Newcastle disease virus of one and seven day old chicks. These results suggest that the vitamin E requirement for broiler breeder birds for maximizing the immune response of chicks may be higher than required for maximizing growth performance.

An important response of the immune system to injury or infection is the production of reactive oxygen species (ROS) and of proinflammatory cytokines such as interleukin-1 (IL-1), interleukin 6 (IL-6) and tumour necrosis factor-α (TNF-α). Reactive oxygen species are produced by macrophages as a respiratory burst which is part of the innate immune response. Macrophages are phagocytic in nature and can bind, engulf and degrade foreign antigens such as bacteria. This effectively and quickly kills invading pathogens without any lag period. Chicken macrophages can kill more than 80% of *Salmonella* cells within 15 minutes (Qureshi *et al.* 1998b). The innate immune system is a very important part of health maintenance as it can react very rapidly to pathogens which enter the body.

However the production of ROS as part of the innate immune response and increased inflammatory cytokine production can in turn cause health problems. There is an adverse alliance between ROS and inflammatory cytokines which can lead to serious tissue damage and poor health. Excessive production of inflammatory cytokines in combination with infection can lead to sepsis, organ failure and rapid muscle protein degradation. In addition, in cells suffering from an inflammatory response have high levels of activated nuclear factor kappa B (NF-κB), a transcription factor that promotes the expression of numerous genes associated with inflammation.

Immune and inflammatory cells are rich in *n*-6 PUFA, especially linoleic and arachidoneic acids. It is possible that an excess dietary supply of these fatty acids could promote or exacerbate the inflammatory response. This may be countered by decreasing the ratio of *n*-6 :*n*-3 PUFA in the feed. This can only be directly achieved by feeding an oil such as fish oil which contains substantial amounts of *n*-3 PUFA.

A considerable amount of work with animals cells and live animals have show that the *n*-3 PUFA from fish oil can alter the production of inflammatory cytokines and reduce the activation of NF-κB (Calder, 2006). The fatty acids, eicosapentanoic acid (EPA) and docosahexanoic acid (DHA), inhibit endotoxin-stimulated production of IL-6 and IL-8 by cultured human epithelial cells. These *n*-3 PUFA can totally abolish up-regulation of TNF-α, IL-1α and IL-1ß in cultured bovine chondrocytes. Eicosapentanoic acid is less potent than arachidonic acid in inducing IL-6 expression in macrophages and prevents NF-κB activation in cultured pancreatic cells. Similarly, EPA or fish oil decreased endotoxin-induced activation of NF-κB in human monocytes.

Animal feeding studies with fish oil support the observations from cell culture work in relation to the effects of long-chain *n*-3 PUFA on NF-κB activation and inflammatory cytokine production. Compared with feeding maize oil, fish oil lowered NF-κB activation in mouse spleen lymphocytes. Feeding fish oil to mice decreases the production of TNF-α, IL-1ß and IL-6 by endotoxin-stimulated macrophages and decreases circulating TNF-α, IL-1ß and IL-6 concentrations in mice injected with endotoxin. Dietary fish oil markedly enhanced the survival of guinea pigs to intraperitoneal endotoxin and reduced the concentrations of circulating TNF-α, IL-1ß and IL-6 concentrations in mice compared to safflower oil.

These observations suggest a range of anti-inflammatory actions of long-chain *n*-3 PUFA. They seem to be able to modify inflammatory gene expression via inhibition of activation of the transcription factor NF-κB. The overall picture that emerges from a range of work on animals is that administration of long chain *n*-3 PUFA in the form of fish oil increases survival on exposure to live pathogens. This is most likely due to an improvement in host immune defences.

It has long been customary to consider the ratio of unsaturated to saturated fatty acids in animal feeds because saturated fatty acids are less well digested than unsaturated fatty acids. This is of particular importance in young animals where efficient digestion of dietary fats and oils is crucial. However from an NbH point of view perhaps feed formulations should also be considered in terms of the ratio of *n*-3 to *n*-6 PUFA. It seems quite possible that the fatty acid composition of a diet will have an important effect upon health maintenance and disease avoidance in animals.

The problem here is that direct supplies of *n*-3 PUFA are only available from fish oils. These are routinely used in fish feeds but not in general monogastric feeds. Some attempts have been made to include linseed oil as a good source of linolenic acid which can be metabolized into *n*-3 PUFA by the animal. However the efficiency of transformation of linolenic to *n*-3 PUFA is very low. Furthermore incorporation of fish oils or linseeed oils also will give potential problems from autoxidation of these materials in the feed.

An alternative strategy may be to reduce the ratio of linoleic to linolenic acid in feeds. The major substrate for production of arachidonic acid and subsequent development of the inflammatory response is linoleic acid. Although linoleic acid is a major fatty acid in soyabean, sunflower and cottonseed oils, other plant oils such as rapeseed, palm or olive oils are much lower in this fatty acid.

Young animals

The initial protection of newly born mammals or newly hatched chicks undoubtedly requires an NbH approach. The milk of mammals and the yolk sac of avian species contain various immunoglobulins and maternal antibodies which protect young animals from infections from pathogens to which the mothers had been exposed during their lives

In newly-hatched chicks the remaining yolk sac contents provide an internal feed for survival during the first days of life, as well as a source of antibodies, until the external feed is taken up. The maximum utilization of the yolk sac contents is therefore very important for the subsequent growth and development of the newly-hatched chick (Mikec *et al.*, 2006). Stresses caused by environmental factors have a negative impact on the development and immunity of the chick. Stress is the principal cause of yolk resorption disorders, which impacts upon the development of the gastrointestinal tract and the health status of the growing chick. The resorption pathway of the yolk sac contents depends upon the energy needs of the chick. If exogenous feed is immediately available the remaining yolk sac contents are poorly resorbed in the under-developed gastrointestinal tract. If there is no feed available, the yolk sac contents enters the blood directly through the yolk sac wall by means of endocytosis which is a more efficient resorption system.

Gastrointestinal immune response

One of the major problems identified with the widespread use of antibiotic growth promoters was the appearance of vancomycin resistant enterococci (VRE) and the subsequent risk of transfer of the infection from animals to humans (Bates *et al.*, 1994). Once an animal is infected with VRE it is very difficult to control it because the organism has such widespread multiple resistance.

An interesting possibility to control gastrointestinal infections with VRE is to elicit an immune response in the gastrointestinal tract by means of an immunostimulatory preparation from dead cells of the bacteria *Enterococcus faecalis* incorporated into the diet (Sakai *et al.*, 2006).

Compared to the control group VRE detection in caeca from birds with the *E. faecalis* treatment was lower on day 14 after the VRE challenge (Table 2). There was also a significant increase in total IgA in the caecal digesta as a result of including the dead *E. faecalis* preparation in the diet.

There are quite intriguing results as working with a dead bacterial preparation is obviously much safer than dosing feed or drinking water with live cultures. Furthermore a dead cell preparation cannot acquire or transmit the vancomycin-resistant plasmid from VRE.

Table 2. Vancomycin-resistant enterococci (VRE) and total IgA in the caecal digesta of broiler chicks.

Parameter measured	*Treatment*	
	Control	*E. faecalis*
Number of chicks	13	13
VRE detection (%)	100	54
VRE numbers (X 10^3 cfu/g)	85.6	8
Total IgA (μg/ml)	284.4	366.1

The mode of action here is probably a stimulation of the local areas in the gastrointestinal tract rather than a systemic immune response. Gram-positive bacteria such as *E. faecalis* are known to stimulate the inflammatory reaction in the mammalian gastrointestinal tract. The relative rapid decline in VRE detection which was manifested as early as three days after challenge suggest the involvement of the innate immune system. However these are initial results and there is a need for further confirmation of this response.

With nutritional measures it is possible to change the immune response in the development of the gastrointestinal tract of the broiler (Rebel *et al.* 2004). Broiler breeders receiving an increased dietary supply of vitamins and trace minerals showed an improved immune response which was carried over to the progeny. For example there was an increased number of day-old chicks descended from breeders which had received high levels of vitamins and minerals. Also the recovery rate from intestinal lesions from malabsorption syndrome was faster for chicks from breeders fed high levels of vitamins and minerals.

Enhanced vaccine response

An extensive programme of vaccination against infectious diseases is widely used in animal production and has given major benefits in terms of improved animal health and resistance to disease. However the immune system of newly hatched chicks is not well developed and this frequently results in poor response to vaccinations and concomitant reduced disease resistance. There is a considerable interest in developing nutritional strategies to improve the response to vaccination in young animals.

The nutricine lutein seems to to increase the efficacy of vaccination to infectious bronchitis virus (Bédécarrats and Leeson, 2006).

Another nutritional strategy to improve immune response is to reduce the ratio of linoleic to linolenic acid in feeds. Linoleic acid is an *n*-6 polyunsaturated fatty acid (PUFA), gives rise to arachidonic acid, and ultimately is proinflammatory by generating increased production of IL-1, TNF-α and IL-6. Linolenic acid and PUFAS from fish oils are *n*-3 fatty acids and limit the proinflammatory response by inhibiting the production of arachdonic acid.

Adding up to 4.39% flaxseed to a poultry feed formulation reduced the linoleic to linolenic acid ratio from 17:1 in the control feed to a low of 2:1 (Puthpongsiriporn and Scheideler, 2005). Feeding these low dietary ratios of linoleic to linolenic acid to newly hatched chicks modified the fatty acid composition of the immune tissues resulting in an increase in antibody production from vaccination against Newcastle disease virus and infectious bursal disease. Reduced ratios of linoleic to linolenic acid also resulted in a decrease in arachidonic acid and increases in EPA and DHA (Table 3).

Table 3. Arachidonic acid, eicosapentanoic acid (EPA) and docosahexanoic acid (DHA) in various immune tissues of pullets (% of total fatty acids).

Pullet age (weeks)	*Ratio in diet (linoleic: linolenic acid)*	*Immune tissue*	*Arachidonic acid*	*EPA*	*DHA*
16	17:1	Spleen	11.47	0.87	1.07
	2:1		6.92	3.29	2.35
16	17:1	Thymus	7.29	0.51	1.14
	2:1		3.63	1.28	2.13
8	17:1	Bursa of Fabricius	9.80	0.05	0.92
	2:1		4.70	0.78	2.68

In general there was approximately a 50% reduction in the proportion of arachidonic acid in the immune tissues when a low linoleic to linolenic acid ratio feed was supplied to the pullets. This change in the ratios of arachidonic acid to EPA and DHA is thought to mediate a more effective immune response through an effect upon eiscosanoid production which in turn resulted in increased antibody production.

These data clearly illustrate that there is an important interaction between an effective response to vaccination and the nutrition of the host. Obviously an important element of NbH would be to ensure that feed formulations are designed to support a good response to vaccination.

Plant-based edible vaccines

It is possible to generate vaccines in transgenic plants and this could be very valuable in an NbH programme for animals as well as for humans (Haq *et al.* 1995).

Vaccine production in transgenic plants has several major advantages compared to classical vaccination use. These include a lower cost because they would be produced from conventional crop husbandry. Also the production of vaccine antigens in plants is highly efficient and relatively small amounts of various crops would be needed for vaccine production. The vaccines would likely be more stable as they would be stored in cells of the host plant, dried and stored at ambient temperatures. This would obviate the necessity of refrigerated storage of vaccines. There is a reduced potential for adverse reactions since the transgenic plant is engineered to express only a small antigenic portion of the pathogen. Such vaccines would also be free from animal pathogens such as prion proteins so there should be no risk of the transfer of animal diseases in these vaccines. There is the potential to generate multicomponent vaccines. The vaccines produced by plant biotechnology are all designed to be orally active (Streatfield *et al.*, 2001). This means that delivery to animals would be simple as the plant containing the vaccine could be simply incorporated into the standard animal feed.

An example of a plant-based edible vaccine is the utilization of the Norwalk virus capsid protein expressed in potatoes as an antigen (Tacket *et al.*, 2000). When the transgenic potatoes were fed to human volunteers 19 of the 20 subjects developed an immune response to the antigen. This confirmed that foreign proteins can be immunogenic when presented to the mucosal immune system via an orally delivered transgenic potato. A multi-component plant-based vaccine comprised of cholera toxin complementary DNAs fused to a rotavirus enterotoxin and enterotoxigenic *Escherichia coli* fimbrae antigen genes was expressed in transgenic potatoes (Yu and Langrióge, 2001). When the transgenic potatoes were used to orally immunize mice there were detectable levels of serum and intestinal antibodies against the pathogen antigens. Diarrhoea symptoms were reduced in severity and duration in passively immunized mouse neonates following rotavirus challenge. Plant-based edible vaccines can offer simultaneous protection against infectious viral and bacterial diseases. Further confirmation of the potential and versatility of plant-based edible vaccines has been provided in studies with hepatitis B surface antigen expressed in transgenic potatoes (Kong *et al.*, 2001). Mice fed the transgenic potatoes produced serum antibodies that exceeded the protective level, and on parenteral boosting, generated a strong long-lasting secondary antibody response. Consumption of transgenic maize engineered to express a gene encoding a subunit of the *E.coli* heat-labile enteroxin gave a rise in the serum IgG anti-enterotoxin in healthy adults (Tacket *et al.*, 2004). Repeated dosing was shown to increase the immune response.

Of more direct relevance to animal health is the production of a vaccine against porcine epidemic diarrhoea virus (PEDV) in transgenic tobacco plants (Bae *et al.*, 2003). This virus is highly contagious and PEDV causes enteritis in pigs at all ages and is often fatal in neonatal piglets. Transgenic tobacco plants were simply lyophilized, ground to a fine powder, suspended in a buffer and fed directly to mice. As shown in Table 4 higher levels of antigen-specific IgA were detected in faecal samples collected from mice fed antigen-expressing transgenic tobacco versus control mice. There was also a dose–response since higher levels of antigen-specific IgA were found in faecal samples of mice fed 5 mg of plant material compared to those fed 1 mg. Feeding mice with a plant-based edible vaccine induced an efficient antigen-specific mucosal immune response.

Table 4. Level of IgA in faecal material specific to the antigen after feeding mice either control or transgenic tobacco.

Amount of antigen	*Control*	*Treatment*
1 mg	0.15	0.30
5 mg	0.24	0.68

IgA was determined using an ELISA system and is expressed as absorbance at 405 nm.

Transgenic lucerne plants have been used to reduce enterotoxigenic *Escherichia coli* (ETEC) excretion in piglets (Joensuu, *et al.*, 2006). The DNA sequence encoding the F4 fimbrial adhesin, FaeG, of ETEC was transformed into edible lucerne plants. By targeting the chloroplasts up to 1% of the total soluble protein fraction of the transgenic lucerne was FaeG. The FaeG in the transgenic plants remained stable for two years when the plant material was dried and stored at room temperature. Administration of the plant-derived FaeG enhanced the immune response against FaeG. The transgenic lucerne plants producing the FaeG subunit protein could be used for production and delivery of oral vaccines against ETEC infections.

Plant-based edible vaccines would be highly desirable for use in animal production. In particular they may offer an enhanced immune response at mucosal sites, including the production of secretory IgA, which serves as a defence against pathogen colonization and infection by preventing the specific interaction of pathogens with mucosal surfaces. There are many important pathogens of animals that cause enteric or respiratory diseases and therefore the mucosal response is an essential first line of defence. Furthermore potential low cost and ease of administration to animals makes this a very attractive concept for an NbH programme.

Conclusions

It is clear that in modern animal production the support of an efficient immune system is extremely important to protect animal health. In particular the innate immune response is critical to disease avoidance in animals since it is a very rapid defence mechanism. In both mammalian and avian species the immune system is influenced by a host of external and internal factors, including environment, genetics, toxins and nutrition. Mycotoxins are well-known immunosuppressors. It is well accepted that nutrition influences the robustness of the immune system but it is still not clear how the various nutrients and nutricines specifically affect the immune system. It is not established whether or not dietary requirements for growth are adequate to support the immune system. Lutein is a good example here where it has little effect upon growth but plays an important role in supporting the immune system. Various non-digestible polysaccharides also have immunomodulating effects. Increasing the ratio of *n*-3 to *n*-6 PUFA in feeds gives benefits in terms of supporting the immune system. Young animals are particularly sensitive to infections from pathogens and good neonatal nutrition is very important for health maintenance and disease avoidance. There is a possibility to improve the immune response to gastrointestinal infections through the use of bacterial cell fragments. Enhanced vaccine response plays an important role in animal health. In particular the development of plant-based edible vaccines will become important here. Their potential low cost and ease of administration to animals makes this a very attractive concept for an NbH programme.

References

Bae, J-L., Lee, J-G., Kang, T-J., Jang, H-S., Jang, Y-S. and Yang, M-S. (2003). Induction of antigen-specific systemic and mucosal immune responses by feeling animals transgenic plants expressing the antigen. Vaccine, 21: 4052-4058.

Bates, J., Jordens, J. Z. and Griffiths, D. T. (1994). Farm animals as a putative reservoir for vancomycin-resistant enterococcal infection in man. Journal of Antimicrobial Chemotherapy, 34: 507-514.

Bédécarrats, G. Y. and Leeson, S. (2006). Dietary lutein influences immune response in laying hens. Poultry Science, 15: 183-189.

Blount, J. D. (2004). Carotenoids and life-history evolution in animals. Archives of Biochemistry and Biophysics, 430: 10-15.

Blount, J. A., Metcalf, N. B., Birkhead, T. R. and Surai, P. F. (2003). Carotenoid modulation of immune function and sexual attractiveness in Zebra finches. Science, 300: 125-127.

Calder, P. C. (2006). Use of fish oil in parenteral nutrition: rationale and reality. Proceedings of the Nutrition Society, 65: 264-277.

Cheng, W., Liu, C-H., Kuo, C-M. and Chen, J. C. (2005). Dietary administration of sodium alginate enhances the immune ability of white shrimp *Litopenaeus vannamei* and its resistance against *Vibrio alginolyticus*. Fish and Shellfish Immunology, 18: 1-12.

Chew, B. P. (1993). Role of the carotenoids in the immune response. Journal of Dairy Science, 76: 2804-2811.

Guo, F. C., Kwakkel, R. P., Williams, B. A., Parmentier, H. K., Li, W. K., Yang, Z. Q. and Verstegen, M. W. A. (2004). Effects of mushroom and herb polysaccharides on cellular and humoral immune responses of *Eimeria tenella*-infected chickens. Poultry Science, 83: 1124-1132.

Hahn, T-W., Lohakare, J. D., Lee, S. L., Moon, W. K. and Chae, B. J. (2006). Effects of supplementation of ß-glucans on growth performance, nutrient digestibility, and immunity in weanling pigs. Journal of Animal Science, 84: 1422-1428.

Haq, T. A., Mason, H. S., Clements, J. D. and Arntzen, C. J. (1995). Oral immunization with a recombinant bacterial antigen produced in transgenic plants. Science, 268: 714-716.

Haq, A-L., Bailey, C. A. and Chinnah, A. (1996). Effect of ß-carotene, lutein, and vitamin E on neonatal immunity of chicks when supplemented in the broiler breeder diets. Poultry Science, 75: 1092-1097.

Huff, G. R., Huff, W. E., Rath, N. C. and Tellez, G. (2006). Limited treatment with ß-1,3/1,6–glucans improves production values of broiler chickens challenged with *Escherichia coli*. Poultry Science, 85: 613-618.

Joensuu, J. J., Verdonck, F., Ehrström, A., Peltola, M., Sijlander-Rasi, H., Nuutila, A. M., Oksman-Caldentey, K. M., Teeri, T. H., Cox, E., Goddeeris, B. M. and Niklander-Teeri, V. (2006). F4 (K88) fimbrial adhesin FaeG expressed in alfalfa reduces F4+ enterotoxigenic *Escherichia coli* excretion in weaned piglets. Vaccine, 24: 2387-2394.

Kim, H. W., Chew, B. P., Wong, T. S., Park, J. S., Weng, B. B. C., Byrne, K. M., Hayek, M. G. and Reinhart, G. A. (2000a). Modulation of humoral and cell-mediated immune responses by dietary lutein in cats. Veterinary Immunology and Immunopathology, 73: 331-341.

Kim, H. W., Chew, B. P., Wong, T. S., Park, J. S., Weng, B. B. C., Byrne, K. M., Hayek, M. G. and Reinhart, G. A. (2000b). Dietary lutein stimulates immune response in the canine. Veterinary Immunology and Immunopathology, 74: 315-327.

Kong, Q., Richter, L., Yang, Y. F., Arntzen, C. J., Mason, H. S. and Thanavala, Y. (2001). Oral immunization with hepatitis B surface antigen expressed in transgenic plants. Proceedings of the National Academy of Science, 98: 11539-11544.

Koutsos, E. A., López, J. C. G. and Klasing, K. C. (2006). Carotenoids from in ovo or dietary sources blunt systemic indices of the inflammatory response in growing chicks (*Gallus gallus domesticus*). Journal of Nutrition, 136: 1027-1031.

Le Floc'h, N., Melchior, D. and Obled, C. (2004). Modification of protein and amino acid metabolism during inflammation and immune system activation. Livestock Production Science, 87: 37-45.

Li, Y. C., Ledoux, D. R., Bermudez, A. J., Fritsche, K. L. and Rottinghaus, G. E. (2000a). Effects of moniliformin on performance and immune function of broiler chicks. Poultry Science, 79: 26-32.

Li, Y. C., Ledoux, D. R., Bermudez, A. J., Fritsche, K. L. and Rottinghaus, G. E. (2000b). The individual and combined effects of fumonisin B_1 and moniliformin on performance and selected immune parameters in turkey poults. Poultry Science, 79: 871-878.

Li, J., Li, D. F., Xing, J. J., Cheng, Z. B. and Lai, C. H. (2006). Effects of ß-glucan extracted from *Saccharomyces cerevisiae* on growth performance, and immunological and somatotropic responses of pigs challenged with *Escherichia coli* lipopolysaccharide. Journal of Animal Science, 84: 2374-2381.

Lowry, V. K., Farnell, M. B., Ferro, P. J., Swaggerty, C. L., Bahl, A. and Kogut, M. H. (2005). Purified ß-glucan as an abiotic feed additive up-regulates the innate immune response in immature chickens against *Salmonella enterica* serovar *Enteritidis*. International Journal of Food Microbiology, 98: 309-318.

Mao, X. F., Piao, X. S., Lai, C. H., Li, D. F., Xing, J. J. and Shi, B. L. (2005). Effects of ß-glucan obtained from the Chinese herb *Astragalus membranaceus* and lipolysaccharide challenge on performance, immunological, adrenal, and somatotropic responses of weanling pigs. Journal of Animal Science, 83: 2775-2782.

Mikec, M., Bidin, Z., Valentic´, A., Savic´ V., Zelenika, A. T., Raguz-Duric´, R. Novak, I. L. and Balenovic M. (2006). Influence of environment and nutritional stressors on yolk sac utilization, development of chicken gastrointestinal system and its immune status. World's Poultry Science Journal, 62: 31-40.

Puthpongsiriporn, U. and Scheideler, S. E. (2005). Effects of dietary ratios of linoleic to linolenic acid on performance, antibody production, and in vitro lymphocyte proliferation in two strains of leghorn pullet chicks. Poultry Science, 84: 846-857.

Qureshi, M. A., Brake, J., Hamilton, P. B., Hagler Jr., W. M. and Nesheim, S. (1998a). Dietary exposure of broiler breeders to aflatoxin results in immune dysfunction in progeny chicks. Poultry Science, 77: 812-819.

Qureshi, M. A., Hussain, I. and Heggen, C. L. (1998b). Understanding immunology in disease development and control. Poultry Science, 77: 1126-1129.

Rebel, J. M. J., van Dam, J. T. P., Zekarias, B., Balk, F. R. M., Post, J., Flores minambres, A. and ter Huurne, A. A. H. M. (2004). Vitamin and trace mineral content in feed of breeders and their progeny: effects of growth, feed conversion and severity of malabsorption syndrome of broilers. British Poultry Science, 45: 201-209.

Sakai, Y., Tsukahara, T., Bukawa, W., Matsubara, N. and Ushida, K. (2006). Cell preparation of *Enterococcus faecalis* strain EC-12 prevents vancomycin-resistant enterococci colonization in the cecum of newly hatched chicks. Poultry Science, 85: 273-277.

Streatfield, S. J., Jilka, J. M., Hood, E. E., Turner, D. D., Bailey, M. R. and Major, J. M. (2001). Plant-based vaccines: unique advantages.

Vaccine, 19: 2742-2748.

Tacket, C. O., Mason, H. S., Losonsky, G., Estes, M. E., Levine, M. M. and Arntzen, C. J. (2000). Human immune responses to a novel norwalk virus vaccine delivered in transgenic potatoes. Journal of Infectious Diseases, 182: 302-305.

Tacket, C. O., Pasetti, M. F., Edelman, R., Howard, J. A. and Streatfield, S. (2004). Immunogenicity of recombinant LT-B delivered orally to humans in transgenic corn. Vaccine, 22: 4385-4389.

Takeda, K., Kaisho, T. and Akira, S. (2003). Toll-like receptors. Annual Review of Immunology, 21: 335-376.

Yu, J. and Langrióge, H. R. (2001). A plant-based multicomponent vaccine protects mice from enteric diseases. Nature Biotechnology, 19: 548-552.

Yun, C-H., Estrada, A., van Kessel, A., Gajadhar, A. A., Redmond, M. J. and Laarveld, B. (1997). ß-(1-3, 1-4) oat glucan enhances resistance to *Eimeria vermiformis* infection in immunosuppressed mice. International Journal for Parasitology, 27: 329-337.

7 Feed-Host Interactions (3) : Oxidative Stress and Disease

Feed has many important roles in animal physiology, one of which is to supply metabolic energy through a series of oxidative reactions of various feed ingredients. Consequently all animals need oxygen for effective production of energy in the mitochondria of cells. However oxygen is also a toxic, mutagenic gas, and excessive oxidation of cellular components leads to a whole spectrum of non-infectious diseases and may exacerbate various infectious diseases. Animals only survive in the presence of oxygen because they have developed various antioxidant defence strategies and because the feed is an important source of antioxidants. Therefore modulation of oxidative stress and of various diseases is the third feed-host interaction.

(1) Maintenance of gastrointestinal integrity
(2) Support of the immune system
(3) Modulation of oxidative stress and disease

During the normal metabolism of nutrients and the respiration processes of animals, oxygen is progressively reduced in the mitochondria to yield water and ATP. However the incomplete reduction of oxygen during this process leads to the formation of chemical entities that have powerful oxidising properties. These are known as reactive oxygen species (ROS) and the basal cellular metabolism in the body of an animal continuously produces ROS.

The maintenance of good vascular tone in the body requires the synthesis of the reactive nitrogen species (RNS), nitrous oxide (NO). This NO is produced from the amino acid arginine by the nitric oxide synthase enzyme and is a common constituent of in the blood of mammals (Rhodes *et al.*, 1995). It may react with other ROS to generate yet more reactive species such as peroxynitirite even in healthy animals. Consequently in normal metabolism there is the continuous production of a plethora of ROS and RNS.

There is of necessity a delicate balance between antioxidants and pro-oxidants in the body. These ROS under normal physiological conditions are controlled by various antioxidant defence mechanisms which include enzymes and antioxidants. Enzymes such as superoxide dismutase converts superoxide radicals to H_2O_2, catalase breaks down H_2O_2 and glutathione peroxidase breaks down peroxides, notably those derived from the oxidation of membrane phospholipids. The ROS can also be neutralised by endogenous antioxidants such as glutathione, vitamin E, vitamin C, and carotenoids.

Increased amounts of ROS are also produced in response to infection as part of a defence response since the ROS are harmful to bacteria. At an infected site in the body there be a local increase in cells of the immune system such as macrophages and polymorphonuclear nutrophils. These release ROS such as superoxide anion ($O_2^{\cdot}$), via the enzyme NADH-oxidase, which leads to the subsequent production of other ROS such as hydrogen peroxide (H_2O_2), hydroxyl radical ($OH^{\cdot}$), and hypochlorous acid (HOCl). These ROS also have the potential to destroy host cells and they have a cytotoxic activity through several different mechanisms such as protein and amino acid oxidation, lipid peroxidation and DNA damage. Lipid oxidative damage leading to the oxidation of thiol groups may alter membrane permeability. The production of aldehyde products such as malondialdehyde and 4-hydroxy-2-nonenal from lipid oxidation may cause modification of proteins. There is also considerable evidence that mycotoxins can be an important stress factor that generates an oxidative stress (Surai and Dvorska, 2005). Mycotoxins may stimulate lipid peroxidation through enhancing free radical production and also they may interfere with the antioxidant defence system of the cell.

Oxidative stress, when ROS accumulate and overwhelm the endogenous antioxidant protection mechanisms in the body, is an important mechanisms for biological damage in live animals (Fellenberg and Speisky, 2006). Lipid peroxidation has been proposed as the principal mechanistic pathway in kidney cell cancer development (Gago-Dominguez and Castelao, 2006). Lipid oxidation and the subsequent onset of oxidative stress may be responsible for an extremely broad spectrum of disease syndromes in humans and animals. These diseases are known as non-infectious, physiological or metabolic diseases. In general they are diet-related and so nutrition plays an important role in controlling and mitigating these diseases.

The gastrointestinal mucosa is constantly exposed to a variety of pro-oxidants derived from ingested food materials. In addition, the mastication and digestion of lipid-containing foods in the gastrointestinal fluids can induce lipid peroxidation due to the exposure of unsaturated lipids to catalytic haem or non-haem iron. Dietary iron remains substantially unabsorbed in the gastrointestinal tract and may support bacterial infection as previously discussed (Chapter 3) and may also be involved in the generation of hydroxyl radicals by a Fenton-type reaction in conjunction with colonic microflora. Phytic acid and its hydrolysis products, which are chelators, exert a protective effect on iron-induced lipid peroxidation (Miyamoto *et al.,* 2000). This raises questions about the effect of using exogenous phytase in animal feeds for the purpose of hydrolysing phytic acid to release available phosphorus. It may be that phytic acid plays a useful role as a natural antioxidant. Therefore supplementation of feeds with exogenous phytase might require further consideration of antioxidant levels in the feed. The natural antioxidant quercetin for example protected rat mucosal intestinal tissues against iron-induced lipid peroxidation (Murota *et al.*, 2004) so alternative antioxidant systems are feasible. This also illustrates the possible benefit of antioxidant nutricines such as quercetin in feed for preventing oxidative damage to the gastrointestinal tract.

Nutrition has a major influence on the pro-oxidant/antioxidant balance in the body and there are numerous potential antioxidant nutricines in feeds. These include vitamins such as C and E, trace minerals such as selenium and zinc as well as other feed components such as carotenoids, anthocyanins and synthetic antioxidants; BHA, BHT and propyl gallate. An adequate dietary intake of antioxidants is important to maintain tissue levels of antioxidants and avoid oxidative stress.

The carotenoids are powerful antioxidants and are able to retard lipid peroxidation by quenching of singlet oxygen and by scavenging of free radicals. Lycopene is the most effective singlet oxygen quencher and free radical scavenger amongst the carotenoids (Shixian *et al.*, 2005). Another common dietary carotenoid lutein, also has significant antioxidant activity. There is increasing evidence that carotenoids act synergistically with other dietary antioxidants such as vitamin E and poylphenols. This again suggest that a wide variety of nutricines will be important in NbH.

There are many materials and compounds derived from plants which have demonstrable antioxidant activities. Animal feeds in general are also based predominantly upon raw materials derived from plants and therefore it should be possible to ensure that the antioxidant level of feeds is adequate. A practical problem here is that adequate antioxidant levels for disease avoidance and health maintenance have not yet been established so feeds cannot be formulated to contain any specific amount of antioxidant activity for NbH.

Oxidative stress and animal health

There have been very successful animal breeding programmes over many years which have led to the introduction of pig and poultry genotypes capable of rapid growth rates and lean muscle deposition coupled with high reproductive performance. However there are also various health issues associated with these new genotypes. One is high mortality in both weaned pigs and sows. Longevity of sows in a sow herd is of major concern in many commercial pig herds. The highest producing and fastest growing animals, both pigs and poultry, may suffer heavy mortalities due to sudden deaths. In weaned piglets and sows the antioxidant capacity is at its lowest with sudden death occurrences (Mahan, 2005).

An oxidative stress in pigs generated by feeding high levels of linseed oil was manifested as increased levels of malondialdehyde in the blood plasma and increased DNA damage in mononuclear blood cells compared to pigs fed starch-supplemented diets (Pajk *et al.*, 2006). Supplementation of the high linoleic acid diets with apples, strawberries or tomatoes significantly decreased the oxidative stress brought about by the linoleic acid. Theses fruits are recognised as having good levels of natural antioxidants. There is increasing interest in supplementing animal feeds with linoleic acid in order to increase the quantity of omega-3 fatty acids in the meat. However this must also be tempered by good antioxidant protection in the feed to avoid an oxidative stress in the animals.

Feeding oxidised oils with high levels of peroxides (754 meq/kg compared to 5 meq/kg in the fresh oil) to female rats during rearing, pregnancy and lactation influenced development of foetuses and suckling pups as well as their antioxidant status and lipid metabolism (Brandsch and Eder, 2004). During the suckling period pups from mothers fed an oxidized oil grew more slowly than pups from mothers fed fresh oil (Figure 1).

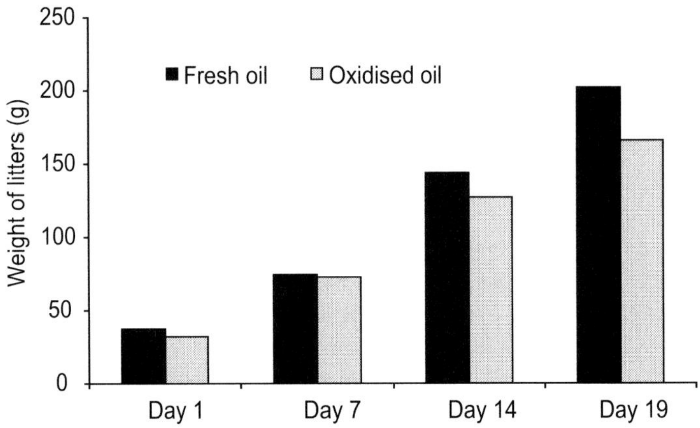

Figure 1. Weight gain of litters of rat pups from dams fed either fresh oil or oxidised oil during the suckling period.

Milk from rats fed the oxidised oil had a lower energy content than milk of rats fed fresh oil (5MJ/kg compared to 7.95 MJ/kg) and also a lower concentration of triacylglycerols (97 mmol/l compared to 204 mmol/l). The possibility of oxidative stress reducing milk quality has important implications for the raising of mammals.

Consumption of oxidized oils by rats also induced neurotoxicity, manifested as pica behaviour, a behaviour characterized by eating a non-feed material such as kaolin and that relates to the degree of discomfort of the animals (Gotoh *et al.*, 2006). Rats fed oil with a peroxide value (PV) of least 138.5 meq/kg consumed significantly more kaolin than the control group. A good quality oil would have a PV of around 5.0 meq/kg. Furthermore rats that consumed oil with a PV of at least 107.2 meq/kg had significantly decreased locomotor activity compared to the control rats. These results suggest that oxidized oils with at least 100 meq/kg PV induced neurotoxicity in the rats.

There is some evidence that the damage caused by mycotoxins is also a form of oxidative stress due to the stimulation of lipid peroxidation in the liver (Rizzo *et al.*, 1994). This may explain the beneficial effect seen with antioxidants such as BHA in mitigating the adverse effects of mycotoxins (Monroe *et al.*, 1986).

In the chick embryo there is considerable metabolism of unsaturated fatty acids which are prone to autoxidation and subsequent oxidative stress. At hatching the chick is suddenly exposed to atmospheric oxygen and has a dramatic increase in metabolic rate. The brain of the day old chick is highly enriched in long chain polyunsaturated fatty acids (C_{20} and C_{22}), and the liver also has a large concentration of unsaturated fatty acids (Surai *et al.*, 1996). It is highly likely that lutein and tocopherol in egg yolk play an important role as antioxidants in reducing oxidative stress during the hatching phase. Lutein contents of eggs in modern poultry production are usually quite low and therefore lutein levels in feeds probably needs to be reconsidered from an animal health point of view.

It is possible to influence the oxidative status of chicks by feeding the breeder hen high levels of antioxidants up to a maximum of 160mg/kg of vitamin E (Lin *et al.*, 2005). The livers and brains of chicks from hens fed the high levels of vitamin E in the breeder diet had lower levels of malondialdehyde, an indicator of lipid peroxidation, and higher levels of antioxidant enzymes, liver catalase and brain superoxide dismutase, than chicks from hens fed low vitamin E levels. These results indicate that maternal supplementation with high levels of vitamin E, from 120-160 mg/kg of feed enhances antioxidative capacity and depresses oxidative stress in chicks.

The avoidance of oxidative stress in cattle is particularly important during critical periods such as the transition from late pregnancy to lactation in dairy cattle and adaptation, relocation and transport in calves and beef cattle (Baldi *et al.*, 2006). Exposure to xenobiotics such as mycotoxins or gossypol or to oxidised fats in feeds may also compromise the antioxidant defence system in the animal.

In the transition period in dairy cattle the total antioxidant capacity of the body is under stress (Bernabucci, *et al.*, 2005). Cows with levels of ß-hydroxybutyrate and nonesterified fatty acids in the blood plasma showed higher levels of ROS and thiobarbituric acid reactive substances

(TBARS) and lower levels of antioxidants. In the transition period cows may suffer an oxidative stress due to the negative energy balance and reduced concentration of many antioxidant nutricines in the blood. A higher oxygen demand for milk synthesis increases the production of ROS within the mammary gland which in turn increases the susceptibility to developing intramammary infections or mastitis.

Major non-infectious diseases

Hypertension and angiotensin converting-enzyme inhibitors

The angiotensin converting-enzyme (ACE) inhibitors are of importance in health since they regulate several systems that influence blood pressure. Angiotensin converting-enzyme converts angiotensin I to angiotensin II which is a potent vasoconstricitor. It also hydrolyzes and inactivates bradykinin, a potent vasodilator. Therefore excessive activity of ACE leads to an increased rate of vasoconstriction and to the development of high blood pressure. This in turn is a risk factor for the development of heart and kidney diseases.

Inhibition of ACE is considered as a first line therapy against hypertension and atherosclerosis and various synthetic inhibitors of ACE are already used in human medicine to reduce hypertension. However the formation of ACE inhibitors by enzymatic hydrolysis of proteins from various food sources has also been reported. These include gelatine, casein from milk, egg and fish proteins. Simulated gastrointestinal digestion of ovalbumin generated several active ACE-inhbitors which had an antihypertensive activity in spontaneously hypertensive rats (Miguel *et al.*, 2006). Enzymatic hydrolyzates of glycinin, the major storage protein of soyabean, have also yielded potent ACE inhibitors (Mallikarjun Gouda *et al.*, 2006). Furthermore this ACE inhibitor from soyabeans was a small pentapeptide comprised of Valine-Leucine-Isoleucine-Valine-Proline, which was resistant to digestion by proteases of the gastrointestinal tract. Consequently there may be an added health benefit from soyabean proteins if the undigested residues act as ACE inhibitors to control blood pressure.

A wide variety of human foods surveyed all showed some ACE inhibiting activity (Actis-Gorette *et al.*, 2006). In this study the inhibition of the ACE was associated with phenolic and flavanol compounds in the food. These groups of nutricines are well recognised as having antioxidant activity and they may exert another important health effect in regulating blood pressure. It is clear that many common feed components may have an ACE inhibiting activity and it may well be that a carefully constructed diet may be important to avoid problems associated with high blood pressure.

Ascites

This is a non-infectious disease in broilers and a major cause of economic losses. It is characterised by hypertrophy of the right ventricle in the heart, a flaccid heart and the accumulation of fluid in the abdominal cavity. The syndrome is a basic problem of oxygen supply and demand that develops in response to cardio-pulmonary insufficiency. Ascites is a multifactorial problem mediated by environmental, nutritional and genetic factors

There has been considerable interest in the relationship between ascites and vitamin E in broilers. Oxidative stress has been implicated in the malfunctioning of mitochondria from lungs of broilers suffering ascites and the syndrome could be alleviated by high levels of dietary vitamin E (Table 1) (Iqbal *et al.*, 2001). Body weights, lung weights and mitochondrial lung protein content in birds suffering from ascites was improved by feeding vitamin E.

Dietary coenzyme $Q_{10,}$ which is a component of the mitochondrial respiratory chain, has a beneficial effect in reducing ascites mortality in broilers (Geng *et al.*, 2004).

A general conclusion is that ascites in broilers is associated with an oxidative stress which is manifested as lung mitochondrial dysfunction. This may be alleviated to some extent by high dietary levels of Vitamin E.

Table 1. Body and lung weights and lung mitochondiral protein content of broilers.

Parameter	*Treatment*			
	Control	*Ascites*	*Vit E** *(no ascites)*	*Vit E** *(with ascites)*
Body weight (kg)	2.49	1.95	2.16	2.30
Lung weight (g)	15.1	12.0	13.5	13.5
Lung mitochondrial protein (mg/mL	12.4	9.4	13.2	13.0

* Vitamin E at 100 I.U./kg feed

Mastitis (intramammary infection)

This is an important economic disease in the dairy industry and it combines infectious and non-infectious disease elements. It is basically an inflammatory reaction in response to bacterial infection of the mammary gland. There is an increased local collection of immune cells such as macrophages and polymorphonuclear neutrophils from the blood into an infected area. The main function of these leukocytes and neutrophils is to engulf pathogens and release ROS to eliminate invading bacteria. The production of ROS however may overwhelm the endogenous antioxidant defences and add to the inflammation causing extensive tissue damage. Supplementation of the diet with exogenous antioxidants may facilitate the cow's recovery from mastitis and protect the secretory epithelial cells.

A model system to study mastitis (Lauzon *et al.,* 2005), involved co-culturing bovine mammary epithelial cells and polymporphonuclear neutrophils. An assay based on the release of the enzyme lactate dehydrogenase was used to indicate cytotoxicity when the epithelial cells were incubated with activated polymorphonuclear neutrophils which caused severe damage to the cells. When the antioxidant, catechin was added to the cultures lactate dehydrogenase release, and thus cell cytotoxicity, was reduced by 77% at 25 μM and by 100% at 50 μM. Glutathione ethyl ester, which is rapidly taken up by cells and then is hydrolyzed to reduced glutathione, also very substantially reduced cell cytotoxicity. These observations strongly suggest that antioxidants such as catechin could be a valuable therapy in various inflammatory diseases such as mastitis. However in later *in vivo* work , with mastitis induced by lipopolysaccharide from *Escherichia coli,* infusion of the antioxidants catechin or glutathione ethyl ester did not exert any protective effect (Lauzon *et al.*, 2006). The infusion of deferoxamine, an iron chelator, decreased milk lactate dehydrogenase suggesting it gave a protective effect against damage induced by the accumulation of polymorphonuclear neutrophils. The use of antioxidants and iron chelators in the treatment of mastitis is certainly worthy of further study as they may reduce the damage in the mammary gland from the inflammatory response. It would also be of value to ascertain whether or not maintaining cows on a diet with a high antioxidant content would assist in avoiding mastitis infections.

An alternative approach to the control of mastitis is to infuse the mammary gland with various antibiotics. However the cure rates obtained with antibiotic therapy is generally poor. Moreover the use of antibiotic in a mastitis treatment programme also poses the risk of antibiotic contamination of milk which is clearly undesirable. The medium chain fatty acid, caprylic acid, which occurs naturally in bovine milk and coconut oil, demonstrated a powerful antibacterial effect against some organisms causing mastitis such as *Streptococcus agalactiae, Strep. dysgalactiae* and *Strep. uberis* (Nair *et al.,* 2005). This offers the possibility of using a nutricine such as caprylic acid as an alternative to antibiotics as an intramammary infusion to treat bovine mastitis.

Retention of foetal membranes (RFM)

This disorder was one of the first conditions to be attributed to depleted antioxidant status. In dairy cows RFM is the cause of endometritis, successive ovarian cycle delay and hence delayed pregnancy resulting in serious economic losses.

There is considerable evidence that oxidative stress was enhanced in animals suffering RFM compared to animals with non-retained placenta. Cows which shed the foetal membranes in <12 hours had higher antioxidant status in the blood plasma than cows which retained the foetal membranes (Miller *et al.*, 1993). Cows with low levels of antioxidants such as alpha-tocopherol and glutathione peroxidase in the blood had higher incidences of RFM than cows with higher antioxidant levels (Campbell and Miller, 1998).

Vitamin A and beta-carotene also have an antioxidant function and they may play a role in preventing RFM. The incidence of RFM was found to be lower in cows supplemented with vitamin A and beta-carotene compared to control animals (Table 2) (Michal *et al.*, 1994). The RFM disorder was lowest in cows supplied with 600 mg beta-carotene per day. A lower dose rate of beta-carotene of 300 mg/day or a vitamin A supplement of 120,000 I.U. per day also significantly reduced the RFM problem. The incidence of metritus was significantly lower in cows supplemented with either 300 mg or 600 mg of bet-carotene and was positively correlated with the incidence of RFM. However vitamin A supplementation did not influence metritus.

Table 2. The influence of beta-carotene and vitamin A on the incidence of retained foetal membrane (RFM) and metritus in dairy cows.

Treatment	*RFM (% of cows)*	*Metritus (% of cows)*
Control	41	18
Beta-carotene (300 mg/day)	33	7
Beta-carotene (600 mg/day)	25	8
Vitamin. A (120,000 I.U./day)	31	15

It seems likely that adequate intakes of vitamin A and beta-carotene were required for the timely release of foetal membranes. Antioxidant requirements of high producing dairy cows may be higher than generally recognized and intakes of antioxidants needed to control the production of ROS may exceed the amounts normally supplied in feeds. This is another example where the levels of nutricines in feeds need to be established in terms of health maintenance and disease avoidance as well as for general growth and productivity.

Lung problems

The lung is a unique tissue in terms of oxidative stress because as opposed to other organs, it is directly exposed to higher oxygen tensions. A typical characteristic of lung diseases is inflammation and activation of inflammatory cells that generate reactive oxygen species (ROS). If lung tissue is exposed to high levels of ROS in an oxidative stress this is likely to have deleterious consequences for lung health.

The lungs are protected against oxidative stress by both antioxidant enzyme systems and small antioxidant molecules. One of the most important enzymes involved in antioxidant defence of the lungs is superoxide dismutase (SOD) which converts superoxide radicals into less harmful hydrogen peroxide. Superoxide is also known to react with nitrous oxide (NO) to produce reactive nitrogen species (RNS), such as peroxynitrite. Therefore SOD has multiple effects in regulating levels of superoxide, hydrogen peroxide and RNS.

The antioxidant status of a diet may be important also in preventing the cytotoxic effect of oxidative stress in lung tissue as well as in the gastrointestinal tract. Several naturally occurring dietary antioxidants including reservatrol, olive leaf polyphenol concentrate and quercetin reduced oxidative stress, as indicated by ROS production, in cultured epithelial lung cells (Table 3) (Zaslaver *et al.*, 2005). Dietary antioxidants may have a useful therapeutic potential in the control and treatment of inflammatory lung diseases.

Table 3. ROS production (arbitrary units) in cytokine stimulated cells treated with resveratrol and olive leaf polypjhenols.

Control	*Cytokine stimulated*	*Resveratrol*	*Olive leaf polyphenols*
90	155	60	50

Calcium status

Calcium is a curious essential element. It is the most abundant mineral element in the animal body. It is a major component of bone and egg shell and a significant component of milk. Consequently it is required in substantial amounts in all diets and therefore an adequate supply of calcium is extremely important for health maintenance and disease avoidance.

After absorption calcium is not freely mobile in the cytoplasm of cells (Trewavas, 1999). Calcium binds to many proteins that are attached to the cytoskeleton or to membrane surfaces. Other important intracellular calcium stores are the endoplasmic reticulum (ER), the mitochondria and possibly the Golgi vesicles. There is some calcium remaining in the cytoplasm after protein binding and organelle uptake known as "resting" calcium. Calcium-dependent calcium-ATPases rapidly pump excess calcium into organelles and vesicles within cells to maintain a low calcium level in the cytoplasm. Calcium channels connect the stores of calcium in the organelles and vesicles with the cytoplasm and permit the flow of calcium between the cytoplasm and the other cellular components. Calcium also plays many important roles in metabolism and is essential for the activity of many enzymes including phospholipase

A_2, nucleases and α-amylase. It is involved in contractile properties of muscle and plays a role in blood clotting.

However the absorption of calcium from the gastrointestinal tract is major problem because many calcium salts are insoluble. A good example is insoluble soaps formed from fatty acids and calcium in the gastrointestinal tract. This should not be a problem in healthy animals but may result in less calcium being available when lipids are malabsorbed. Oxalic acid and phytic acids, both of which occur in feed raw materials form insoluble complexes with calcium and this may inhibit absorption. Dietary fibre may also bind calcium although microbial fermentation in the large intestine may well release this calcium and it would become available again.

Various compounds such as lactose, gastric acids, bile acids and the active form of vitamin D_3 (1,25-dihydroxycholecalciferol) improve calcium absorption in the small intestine. Lactose, which is the major carbohydrate in milk, stimulates the absorption of calcium by interacting with the absorptive cells of the gastrointestinal tract to increase their permeability to calcium (Armbrecht and Wasserman, 1976). In the stomach some calcium is probably converted into the more soluble chloride form by reaction with hydrochloric acid. In the small intestine calcium may be kept in solution by reaction with bile acids. This may also be a beneficial effect of the use of organic acids in animal feeds, particularly in piglet diets and in layer rations. The presence of acid in the gastrointestinal tract should ensure that calcium is readily absorbed but this requires further investigation.

It seems that various non-digestible oligosaccharides have a general effect in stimulating calcium absorption (Van Loo *et al.*, 1999, Scholz-Ahrens and Schrezenmeir, 2002). Non-digestible oligosaccharides are readily fermented by bacteria in the large intestine and this increases volatile fatty acid and lactic acid production. This would in turn increase calcium solubility in the large intestine. Therefore improved calcium absorption in the large intestine may be related to this fatty acid production. This introduces a new concept as it is generally accepted that calcium absorption occurs mainly in the small intestine.

Rats fed on a diet containing galactooligosaccharides absorbed calcium more efficiently than those on the control diet and had an improved calcium retention (Table 4) (Chonan and Watanuki, 1995). The bone ash weight and tibia calcium content of rats fed on galactooligosaccharides was significantly higher than those of control animals (Chonan *et al.*, 1995). Other non-digestible oligosaccharides such as fructooligosaccharides also enhance calcium absorption (Morohashi *et al.*, 1998), so the response is likely to be a general effect of non-digestible oligosaccharides.

Table 4. Effect of galactooligosaccharides (GOS) on the apparent calcium absorption and retention in rats.

Calcium uptake	*Treatment*		
	Control	*GOS (5%)*	*GOS (10%)*
Absorption (%)	72.0	81.7	86.3
Retention (%)	71.9	81.5	86.1

Various non-digestible oligosaccharides have been widely studied as prebiotics but now it is interesting to think of these materials perhaps as helping in the difficult task of calcium absorption. Feeding of various non-digestible oligosaccharides might have a useful benefit in improving bone calcification and consequently various skeletal problems of animals..

Calcium plays a central role in oxidative stress through its' effects upon mitochondria. (Crawford *et al.,* 1998). Oxidative stress leads to a release of calcium from intracellular endoplasmic reticular and mitochondrial stores. This calcium release results in an elevation of cytosolic levels which has been linked to cellular damage, activation of mitochondrial permeability transition protein (MPT), growth arrest and disease. Calcium may also be responsible for activating nucleases that directly degrade the mitochondrial RNA and DNA. Activation of calcium–dependent nucleases is a known consequence of cellular stress. There is a general calcium-dependent degradation of mitochondrial polynucleotides following exposure to oxidative stress. This suggests that an early response to oxidative stress would be a dramatic decline in mitochondrial biosynthesis.

Calcium nutrition is of major importance for all species of animals. It has evident welfare effects as well as serious implications for the economics of growth, lactation and egg production. Dietary calcium also plays a key role in the regulation of energy metabolism and obesity (Zemel and Miller, 2004). Increasing dietary calcium without restricting energy appears to cause a repartitioning of dietary energy from adipose tissue to lean body mass which results in a net reduction in fat mass. This has been observed experimentally in both rats and mice. This may be of relevance in the feeding of sows and of poultry breeding stock where weight gains need to be restricted in order to maintain maximum productivity.

Restriction of feed intake in broiler breeder hens to 50-60% of *ad libitum* is an effective and practical management system to reduce various non-infectious diseases and to improve production (Chen *et al.,* 2006). If broiler breeders are allowed feed *ad libitum* during the rearing period they undergo sexual maturation and begin laying eggs earlier than feed- restricted birds and then exhibit a drop in production at an earlier age and ultimately produce fewer eggs. Birds fed *ad libitum* also have significantly increased body fat and in effect will become obese. It is interesting to speculate that improvement in calcium nutrition might reduce weight gain in broiler breeders without drastic feed restriction. This would have useful welfare implications.

Assessment of calcium requirement is not easy and the concept of maximal calcium retention has been used as a functional indicator of calcium requirement in humans (Cashman and Flynn, 1999) and this could also be of relevance in animal nutrition. To achieve maximum skeletal strength it is important to develop and maintain a calcium reserve in the skeleton which depends upon an adequate calcium intake. Maximum calcium retention is achieved at a level of calcium nutrition where bone growth is maximized but this is not readily measured in farm animals. However at calcium intakes above the maximum requirement calcium may be absorbed but instead of being retained in the skeleton it is excreted in the urine and this could readily be measured.

Bone and joint problems

Bone is a very complex material. It consists of collagen fibres, a mineral component as crystals of calcium and phosphate in the form of hydroxyapatite ($Ca_{10}(PO_4)_6(OH)_2$ and other ions and a ground substance formed by glycoproteins. There are two morphologically different forms of bone in the skeleton. These are cortical (compact) and cancellous or trabecular (spongy) bone. Cortical bone is dominant in the femur and tibia whereas spongy bone is dominant in the vertebrae and pelvis. Cortical bone provides rigidity and is mainly responsible for mechanical and protective functions. Spongy bone provides elasticity. It is metabolically more active than cortical bone and is responsible for approximately 50% of skeletal metabolism.

Bone is a living tissues which undergoes a continuous cycle of bone formation, involving osteocyte and osteoblast cells, and bone resorption involving osteoclasts. In healthy adult animals the activities of these cells are normally coupled so that no marked net increase or decrease in bone mass occurs. However with bone diseases such as osteoporosis, bone turnover re-modelling is markedly increased and the activities of these cells are no longer coupled. Osteoclast activity dominates over osteoblast activity and a marked net increase in bone loss occurs.

Despite efforts to improve calcium nutrition in animals, a major source of non-infectious disease is related to problems of bone structure and skeletal development. In particular leg disorders of broilers are important welfare and economic issues in the poultry industry (Waldenstedt, 2006). The rapid growth rates of animals raised for food and which requires rapid deposition of muscle tissue, frequently exceeds the capacity of the skeleton to support the animal. This is manifested in various bone and joint problems such as lameness in pigs and cattle, tibial dyschondroplasia and other leg weaknesses in broilers, tendon strain and damage in horses. A disease known as nutritional degenerative myopathy can occur in cattle on pasture in the spring. This is characterised by skeletal and cardiac problems leading to lameness and sometimes to sudden death (Walsh *et al.*, 1993) and antioxidant status of the animals seems to be important here.

The skeleton is extremely important in protecting the internal organs such as the brain, spinal cord, heart and lungs. It is the attachment site for muscles and ligaments and supports movement of the body. The skeleton is also a metabolic reservoir for calcium, phosphorus and other minerals. Poultry in particular have developed a specific type of bone, medullary bone, which can be quickly formed and resorbed in response to the extreme demand for calcium during egg laying. This medullary bone in avian species enables birds to store large amounts of calcium that is readily available to meet the demands of egg shell formation. Bone is also an important source of calcium for foetal development and for milk synthesis in lactating dairy cows.

Adequate bone development requires a certain amount of physical activity as well as good nutrition. It has long been known that vitamins C and D are very important for bone formation and animal diets must certainly be well supplied with these vitamins to avoid bone and joint problems. Most feed raw materials are very poor in vitamin D and therefore this vitamin is usually added to feeds as vitamin D_3 (1,25-dihydroxycholecalciferol). For broilers up to 14 days of age vitamin D_3 requirements may be in the range of 35-50 μg/kg of feed for cortical bone quality (Whitehead *et al.*, 2004). These requirements are much higher than previous estimates and may be related to the higher calcium requirements of modern broiler genotypes.

The long-term feeding of various lipids altered the mature bone ash content, collagen and cross links levels in Japanese quail (Liu *et al.*, 2004). There were significant decreases in the amounts of bone mineral and collagen cross links in Quail fed soyabean oil or chicken fat compared to those consuming fish oil or hydrogenated soyabean oil. This was probably related to increased production of prostaglandin E_2 production in birds fed soyabean oil or chicken fat and this in turn is related to the higher amounts of omega-6 PUFAs which would be found in the soyabean oil and chicken fat diets.

The lipoxygenase enzyme has been implicated in skeletal development (Klein *et al.*, 2004). Lipoxygenases catalyze the oxygenation of unsaturated fatty acids and have been implicated in the pathogenesis of many disease such as, atherosclerosis, asthma and cancer. However it also appears that lipoxygensases may have negative effects upon skeletal development. The use of chemical inhibitors of lipoxygenase improved bone density and strength in mice used as models for osteoporosis. Furthermore oxidized lipids inhibit osteoblast differentiation and bone formation. Again good antioxidant status in animals will have multiple health benefits.

Lactoferrin, is an iron-binding glycoprotein which occurs naturally in milk. It is also produced by many exocrine glands and is an important constituent in neutrophils. Its' action as an iron chelator may also give it a role as an antimicrobial agent as discussed in Chapter 3. However physiological concentrations of lactoferrin have also been shown to stimulate mitogenesis, differentiation and survival of the bone-forming cells, osteoblasts, (Cornish *et al.*, 2005). It also decreases the formation of bone-resorbing cells, osteoclasts. It is likely that lactoferrin has a physiological role in skeletal development. It may have potential as a nutricine to alleviate or to avoid bone disorders such as osteoporosis and it might have value as a local agent to promote bone repair.

The aetiology of joint and bone problems is generally quite complex and is influenced by many different factors such as genetics, management, nutrition, hygiene and other disease syndromes. Bacterial, viral and parasitic infections in the gastrointestinal tract which decrease nutrient absorption and the presence of anti-nutritional factors in the feed may also induce joint and bone problems.

Oxidative stress and infectious diseases

Oxidative stress is also becoming increasingly implicated in the onset of infectious diseases. This has already been discussed in terms of modifying the virulence of *Coxsackievirus* (Beck *et al.*, 1994) (Chapter 3), but ROS may also be involved in the pathogenesis of several viral diseases (Peterhans, 1997). The ROS are key participants in damage caused by viral infection such as inflammation of epithelial cells and they have been implicated in the pathogenesis of influenza (Peterhans *et al.*, 1987; Hennet *et al.*, 1992).

Oxidative mechanisms have been shown to be important in the development of influenza in mice (Hennet *et al.*, 1992). Infection of mice with influenza virus resulted in a decrease in the total concentration of the antioxidants glutathione, vitamins C and E in the lungs and liver. In particular changes in the concentrations of antioxidants in the liver were noticed in the early stages of infection. In addition ROS produced in the lungs may inactivate protease inhibitors which leads to a increase in infectivity of the influenza virus.

In another study when mice were infected intranasally with influenza virus, systemic effects of the infection were dramatic, culminating in death after five or six days (Hayek *et al.*, 1997). Cells lavaged out of the lungs of infected mice showed an increased production of singlet oxygen and a reduced concentration of the antioxidants alpha-tocopherol, ascorbate and glutathione. Changes in the concentrations of antioxidants in the liver were also noticed in the early stages of infection and this may reduce the ability of the animals to resist an oxidative stress and exacerbate the generation of ROS. Supplementation with excess vitamin E (500 ppm for 6 weeks) of old mice reduced influenza lung titers 25-fold when compared with mice fed the control diet Young mice responded less dramatically but five days after infection still showed a 15-fold reduction in virus titers in lung tissue. In this instance high levels of antioxidant nutricines exerted a therapeutic effect and reduced the amount of virus in the tissues. These observations suggest that infection was associated with an oxidative stress and in the light of current concerns about avian influenza they maybe quite important. It is would certainly be interesting to ascertain whether or not significant levels of dietary antioxidants would assist in the resistance of animals to viral diseases.

Newcastle disease virus (NVD) is an important poultry pathogen and the antioxidant BHT has been demonstrated to prevent mortality in chickens exposed to this virus (Brugh, 1977). Inclusion of BHT in poultry diets seems to protect chickens against NVD infection (Brugh, 1984). In a study with purified NVD, BHT caused a 92% reduction in infectivity (Winston *et al.*, 1980). Electron microscopy of the BHT-treated virus particles revealed damage to the envelope of the particle suggesting that BHT may have a direct antiviral effect in this instance.

Conclusions

During normal metabolism there is always the production of reactive oxygen species (ROS) and reactive nitrogen species (RNS). These are kept under control by a range of antioxidant enzymes and antioxidant molecules in the body. An oxidative stress develops when the ROS and RNS accumulate and overwhelms the endogenous antioxidant protection mechanisms in the body. This may in turn lead to the development of a wide range of both non-infectious and infectious disease syndromes. Nutrition has a major influence upon the pro-oxidant/antioxidant balance in the body and there are numerous potential antioxidant nutricines in feeds. Oxidative stress has serious effects upon animal health and can cause increased DNA damage, affect foetal development, induce neurotoxicity and increase the susceptibility to mastitis. There are several important non-infectious diseases in animals; hypertension, ascites, mastitis, retention of foetal membranes, lung problems, calcium status, and bone and joint problems, which are influenced by oxidative stress. Oxidative stress also plays a role in the onset of some infectious diseases, particularly those of viral origin and antioxidant status of the animals may be important here. Antioxidant nutricines are certainly important components of an NbH strategy as they influence so many factors related to health.

References

Actis-Goretta, L., Ottaviani, J. I. and Frage, C. G. (2006). Inhibition of angiotensin converting enzyme activity by flavanol-rich foods. Journal of Agricultural and Food Chemistry, 54: 229-234.

Armbrecht, H. J. and Wasserman, R. H. (1976). Enhancement of Ca^{++} uptake by lactose in the small intestine. Journal of Nutrition, 106: 1265-1271.

Baldi, A., Pinotti, L. and Fusi, E. (2006). Influence of antioxidants on ruminant health-a review. Ruminants, Society of Feed Technologists, April, UK.

Beck M. A., Kolbeck P. C., Rohr L. H., Shi Q., Morris V. C. and Levander, O. A., (1994) Increased virulence of a human enterovirus (coxsackievirus B3) in selenium-deficient mice. Journal of Infectious Diseases, 170: 351-357.

Bernabucci, U., Ronchi, B., Lacetera, N. and Tardone, A. (2005). Influence of body condition score on the relationships between metabolic status and oxidative stress in periparturient dairy cows. Journal of Dairy Science, 88: 2017-2026.

Brandsch, C. and Eder, K. (2004). Effects of peroxidation products in thermoxidised dietary oil in female rats during rearing, pregnancy and lactation on their reproductive performance and the antioxidative status of their offspring. British Journal of Nutrition, 92: 267-275.

Brugh, M. Jr. (1977). Butylated hydroxytoluen protects chickens exposed to Newcastle disease virus. Science, 197: 1291-1292.

Brugh, M. (1984). Effects of feed additives and feed contaminants on the susceptibility of chickens to viruses. Progress in Clinical and Biological Research, 161: 229-234.

Campbell, M. H. and Miller, J. K. (1998). Effect of supplemental dietary vitamin E and zinc on reproductive performance of dairy cows and heifers fed excess iron. Journal of Dairy Science, 81: 2693-2699.

Cashman, K. D. and Flynn, A. (1999). Optimal nutrition: calcium, magnesium and phosphorus. Proceedings of the Nutrition Society, 58: 477-487.

Chen, S. E., McMurty, J. P. and Walzem, R. L. (2006). Overfeeding-induced ovarian dysfunction in broiler breeder hens is associated with lipotoxicity. Poultry Science, 85: 70-80.

Chonan, O. and Watanuki, M. (1995). Effect of galactooligosaccharides on calcium absorption in rats. Journal of Nutritional Science and Vitaminology, 41: 95-104.

Chonan, O., Matsumoto, K. and Watanuki, M. (1995). Effect of galactooligosaccharides on calcium absorption and preventing bone loss in ovariectomized rats. Bioscience, Biotechnology and Biochemistry, 59: 236-239.

Crawford, D. R., Abramova, N. E. and Davies, K. J. A. (1998). Oxidative stress causes a general, calcium dependent degradation of mitochondrial polynucleotides. Free Radical Biology and Medicine, 25: 1106-1111.

Cornish, J., Grey, A. B., Naot, D., Palmano, K. P., Haggarty, N. W., Callon, K. E. and Reid, I. R. (2005). Lactoferrin and bone: an overview of recent progress. Australian Journal of Dairy Technology, 60: 53-57.

Fellenberg, M. A. and Speisky, H. (2006). Antioxidants: their effect on broiler oxidative stress and its meat oxidative stability. World's Poultry Science Journal, 62: 53-76.

Gago-Dominguez, M. and Castelao, J. E. (2006). Lipid peroxidation and renal cell carcinoma: further supportive evidence and new mechanistic insights. Free Radical Biology and Medicine, 40: 721-733.

Geng, A. L., Guo, Y. M. and Yang Y. (2004). Reduction of ascites mortality in broilers by coenzyme Q_{10}. Poultry Science, 83: 1587-1593.

Gotoh, N., Watanabe, H., Osato, R., Inagaki, K., Iwasawa, A and Wada, S. (2006). Novel approach on the risk assessment of oxidized fats and oils for perspectives of food safety and quality. I. Oxidized fats and oils induces neurotoxicity relating pica behavior and hypoactivity. Food and Chemical Toxicology, 44: 493-498.

Hayek M. G., Taylor S. F., Bender B. S., Han S. N., Meydani M., Smith D. E., Eghtesada S. and Meydani S. N. (1997). Vitamin E supplementation decreases lung virus titers in mice infected with influenza. Journal of Infectious Diseases, 176: 273-276.

Hennet, T., Peterhans, E. and Stocker, R. (1992). Alterations in antioxidant defences in lungs and liver of mice infected with influenza A virus. Journal of General Virology, 73: 39-46.

Iqbal, M., Cawthon, D., Wideman Jr., R. F. and Bottje W. G. (2001). Lung mitochondrial dysfunction in pulmonary hypertension syndrome. II. Oxidative stress and inability to improve function with repeated additions of adenosine diphosphate. Poultry Science, 80: 656-665.

Klein, R. F., Allard, J., Avnur, Z., Nikolcheva, T., Rotstein, D., Carlos, A. S., Shea, M., Waters, R. V., Belknap, J. K., Peltz, G. and Orwoll, E. S. (2004). Regulation of bone mass in mice by the lipoxygenase gene *Alox15*. Science, 303: 229-232.

Lauzon, K., Zhao, X., Bouetard, A., Delbecchi, L., Paquette, B. and Lacasse, P. (2005). Antioxidants to prevent bovine neutrophil-induced mammary epithelial cell damage. Journal of Dairy Science, 88: 4295-4303.

Lauzon, K., Zhao, X., and Lacasse, P. (2006). Deferoxamine reduces tissue damage during endotoxin-induced mastitis in dairy cows. Journal of Dairy Science, 89: 3846-3857

Lin, Y-F., Tsai, H-L., Lee, Y-C. and Chang, S-J. (2005). Maternal vitamin E supplementation affects the antioxidant capability and oxidative stress of hatching eggs. Journal of Nutrition, 135: 2457-2461.

Liu, D., Veit, H. P. and Denbow, D. M. (2004). Effects of long-term dietary lipids on mature bone mineral content, collagen, crosslinks and prostaglandin E_2 production in Japanese quail. Poultry Science, 83: 1876-1883.

Mahan, D. (2005). Feeding the sow and piglet to achieve maximum antioxidant and immunity protection. In: Re-defining mineral nutrition Eds: Talor-Pickard, J. A. and Tucker, L. A. J. Nottingham University Press, Nottingham; UK, pp. 63-73.

Mallikarjun Gouda, K. G., Gowda, L. R., Appu Rao, A. G. and Prakash, V. (2006). Angiotensin I-converting enzyme inhibitory peptide derived from glycinin, the 11S globulin of soybean (*Glycine max*). Journal of Agricultural and Food Chemistry, 54: 4568-4573.

Michal, J. J., Heirman, L. R., Wong, T. S., Chew, B. P., Frigg, M. and Volker, L. (1994). Modulatory effects of dietary ß-carotene on blood and mammary leukocyte function in peripartum dairy cows. Journal of Dairy Science, 77: 1408-1421.

Miguel, M., Aleixandre, M. M., Ramos, M. and López-Fandiño, R. (2006). Effect of simulated gastrointestinal digestion on the antihypertensive properties of ACE-inhibitory peptides derived from ovalbumin. Journal of Agricultural and Food Chemistry, 54: 726-731.

Miller, J. K., Brzezinska-Slebodzinska, E. and Madsen, F. C (1993). Oxidative stress, antioxidants, and animal function. Journal of Diary Science, 76: 2812-2823.

Miyamoto S., Kuwata G., Imai M., Nagao A. and Terao J. (2000). Protective effect of phytic acid hydrolysis products on iron-induced lipid peroxidation of liposomal membranes. Lipids, 35: 1411-1413.

Monroe D. H., Holeski C. J., and Eaton D. L. (1986). Effects of single-dose and repeated-dose pre-treatment with 2(3)-tert-butyl-4-hydroxyanisole (BHA) on the hepatobiliary disposition and covalent binding to DNA of aflatoxin B_1 in the rat. Food and Chemical Toxicology, 24: 1273-1281.

Morohashi, T., Sano, T., Ohta, A. and Yamada, S. (1998). True calcium absorption in the intestine is enhanced by fructooligosaccharide feeding in rats. Journal of Nutrition, 128: 1815-1818.

Murota K., Mitsukuni Y., Ichikawa M., Tsushida T., Miyamoto S. and Terao J. (2004). Quercetin-4'-glucoside is more potent than quercetin-3-glucoside in protection of rat intestinal mucosa homogenates against iron-induced lipid peroxidation. Journal of Agricultural and Food Chemistry, 52: 1907-1912.

Nair, M. K. M., Joy, J., Vasudevan, P., Hinckley, L., Hoagland, T. A. and Venkitanarayanan. K. S. (2005). Antibacterial effect of caprylic acid and monocaprylin on major bacterial mastitis pathogens. Journal of Dairy Science, 88: 3488-3495.

Pajk, T., Rezar, V., Levart, A. and Salobir, J. (2006). Efficiency of apples, strawberries, and tomatoes for reduction of oxidative stress in pigs as a model for humans. Nutrition, 22: 376-384.

Peterhans E., Grob M., Bürge T. and Zanoni R. (1987). Virus-induced formation of reactive oxygen intermediates in phagocytic cells. Free Radical Research Communications, 3: 39-46.

Peterhans E. (1997). Oxidants and antioxidants in viral diseases: Disease mechanisms and metabolic regulation. Journal of Nutrition, 127: 962S-965S.

Rhodes, P. M., Leone, A. M., Francis, P. L., Struthers, A. D. and Moncada, S. (1995). The L-arginine: nitric oxide pathway is the major source of plasma nitrite in fasted humans. Biochemical and Biophysical Research Communications, 209: 590-596.

Rizzo R. F., Atroshi F., Ahotupa M., Sankari S.and Elovaara E. (1994) Protective effect of antioxidants against free radical-mediated lipid peroxidation induced by DON or T-2 toxin. Journal of Veterinary Medicine, A 41: 81-90.

Scholz-Ahrens, K. E. and Schrezenmeir, J. (2002). Inulin, oligofructose and mineral metabolism-experimental data and mechanism. British Journal of Nutrition, 87, Suppl. 2: S179-S186.

Shixian, Q., Dai, Y., Kakuda, Y., Shi, J., Mittal, G., Yeung, D. and Jiang, Y. (2005). Synergistic anti-oxidative effects of lycopene with other bioactive compounds. Food Reviews International, 21: 295-311.

Surai P. F., Noble R. C. and Speake B. K. (1996). Tissue-specific differences in antioxidant distribution and susceptibility to lipid peroxidation during development of the chick embryo. Biochimica et Biophysica Acta, 1304: 1-10.

Surai, P. F. and Dvorska, J. E. (2005). Effects of mycotoxins on antioxidant status and immunity. *In*: The Mycotoxin Blue Book. *Ed:* D. E. Diaz. Nottingham University Press, Nottingham, UK pp.93-137.

Trewavas, A. (1999). Le calcium, c'est la vie: calcium makes waves. Plant Physiology, 120: 1-6.

Van Loo, J., Cummings, J., Delzenne, N., Englyst, H., Franck, A., Hopkins, M., Kok, N., Macfarlane, G., Newton, D., Quigley, M., Roberfroid, M., van Vliet, T. and van den Heuvel, E. (1999). Functional food properties of non-digestible oligosaccharides: a consensus report from the ENDO project (DGX11 AIR11-CT94-1095). British Journal of Nutrition, 81: 121-132.

Waldenstedt, L. (2006). Nutritional factors of importance for optimal leg health in broilers: A review. Animal Feed Science and Technology, 126: 291-307.

Walsh, D.M., Kennedy, S., Blanchflower, W.J., Goodall, E.A. and Kennedy, D.G. (1993). Vitamin E and selenium deficiencies increase indices of lipid peroxidation in muscle tissue of ruminant calves. International Journal of Vitamin and Nutritional Research, 63: 188-194.

Whitehead, C.C., McCormak, H.A., McTier, L. and Fleming, R.H. (2004). High vitamin D_3 requirements in broilers for bone quality and prevention of tibial dyschondroplasia and interactions with dietary calcium, available phosphorus and Vitamin A. British Poultry Science, 45: 425-436.

Winston, V. D., Bolen, J. B. and Consigli, R. A. (1980). Effect of butylated hydroxytoluene on Newcastle disease virus. American Journal of Veterinary Research, 41: 391-394.

Zaslaver, M., Offer, S., Kerem, Z., Stark, A. H., Weller, J. I., Eliraz, A. and Madar, Z. (2005). Natural compounds derived from foods modulate nitric oxide production and oxidative status in epithelial lung cells. Journal of Agricultural and Food Chemistry, 53: 9934-9939.

Zemel, M. B. and Miller, S. L. (2004). Dietary calcium and dairy modification of adiposity and obesity risk. Nutrition Reviews, 62: 125-131.

8 Feed Intake and Health Assessment

An appropriate intake of both nutrients and nutricines will obviously be important in an NbH strategy. Moreover it would be desirable from both production and scientific points of view if animal health could be routinely assessed and monitored during the production cycle and related to feed intake. This would indicate whether or not appropriate strategies were being used. However whilst feed intake is routinely measured in many instances in practice, measurement or assessment of health is extremely complex and routine procedures are not yet readily available.

The word "health" in itself is difficult to define precisely in scientific terms as it generally connotes a state of well-being. It is also frequently perceived in a negative fashion as the absence of disease but this again is very difficult to measure. Health and disease are both due to a combination of gene expression and metabolic responses to a pathogen or to the environment, which are themselves influenced by nutrients and nutricines. This can lead to the development of infectious diseases and non-infectious diseases or to good health. Consequently it is extremely difficult to objectively measure health, particularly in animals which are not evidently sick or ill. Despite these difficulties the overall objective of modern animal nutrition must be to efficiently raise healthy animals.

Feed intake

Feed intake is an extremely important parameter in animal nutrition. Feed is usually the most expensive input in animal production often accounting for up to 70% of total inputs. Therefore it is very important that the animals consume adequate amounts of high quality feed to maximise their productivity. Conversely a reduction of expected feed intake is often an indication of health problems. This may be due to subclinical infections that leads to no visible symptoms, but where overall performance is reduced, or to serious pathogen challenge of the animals leading to the onset of clinical disease.

The response of animals to the intake of nutrients and nutricines in feed is usually measured in economically important outputs such as body weight gain, breast meat yield, egg output, milk production or feed conversion efficiency depending upon the species of interest. Clearly these will also depend upon good animal health. Therefore it is of interest not to think of nutrient requirements but rather on nutritional responses (Gous, 2006). The real need is to know how populations of animals raised for food respond to increasing dietary levels of the various nutrients and nutricines. Important health criteria for animals are also flock uniformity and mortality.

The mechanism underlying the reduction in feed intake during a pathogen challenge is not clear but is probably largely due to an effect on appetite. This is most likely related to the production of various cytokines in response to the pathogen challenge. A general model has been developed to predict feed intake during pathogen challenge (Sandberg *et al.*, 2006). This uses the concept of relative feed intake (RFI) which is defined as the feed intake (kg/d) of the animal challenged by a pathogen divided by its feed intake in the same state had it not been challenged. Monitoring feed intake is probably one of the most useful parameters by which to assess animal health.

Feed intake and NbH in early life

The environment encountered during foetal life and in the neonatal stages appears to be strongly related to the incidence of non-infectious diseases in later life (Langley-Evans, 2006). The level of nutrition during gestation and neonatal periods has a great influence upon the subsequent development and health status of the adult animal. This system whereby events in early life trigger permanent responses in later life have been described as nutritional or metabolic programming (Lucas, 1991). This describes the process whereby a stimulus or insult in early life produces long-term changes in tissue structure or function. Programming is the consequence of the innate capacity of developing tissues to adapt to the conditions that prevail during early life, which for almost all cell types in all organs is an ability that is present for only a short period before birth.

This concept has been described as "the developmental origins of health and disease hypothesis" (Langley-Evans, 2006). It was originally developed to explain association between patterns of foetal and infant growth and major disease states in human populations, but has received strong support from experimental studies in animals.

Nutritional programming has been extensively studied in various animal species including, rat, mouse, guinea-pig, sheep and pigs. It has been consistently noted that one aspect of foetal exposure to any form of under-nutrition is elevated blood pressure. Studies with larger animals such as sheep suggest that programming of cardiovascular function also occurs in all animals. . These studies have all demonstrated that variation in the quality or quantity of nutrient provision during gestation and lactation have a major impact upon tissue development and function and can both promote disease susceptibility or health maintenance (Langley-Evans, 2004). Clearly maternal and neonatal nutrition has a huge impact upon subsequent health and growth of the animals in later life and will be of enormous importance in NbH.

Nutritional requirements

The purpose of adequate nutrition must be to achieve optimum growth and health of the animals being raised for food. However what constitutes an adequate and appropriate diet for animals is not easily defined. Dietary recommendations are usually based on nutrient intakes rather than feed intakes and many factors affect the overall value of a given amount of feed. Intake of feed also inevitably brings with it intake of a wide variety of nutricines which are rarely considered. Environmental conditions, physiological state and genetic origin will also influence the nutritional requirement and the ability to utilize feeds efficiently.

There has been tremendous progress in the nutritional sciences over the last century so that now in the early 21st Century all the required or essential nutrients including vitamins, fatty acids and amino acids are known. The types and amounts of the various nutrients to support good animal growth are fairly well established. The availability of the various nutrients supplied by different feeds, and the effect of feed manufacturing processes on these nutrients has been thoroughly studied. Nevertheless there are still problems of bioavailability, of nutrient-nutrient and nutrient-nutricine interactions. This large amount of nutritional work that has been undertaken has led to the development of nutritional standards for animals where the minimum amounts of various nutrients required to avoid deficiency symptoms has been established.

In current nutritional research, new functions and new roles for nutrients and nutricines in disease prevention and health promotion are being discovered. The functions and requirements of feed are becoming ever-more extensive and it is far less well understood whether the general nutritional requirements established for growth and maintenance of body weight are equally suitable for disease avoidance, development of the immune system, and maintenance of health and well-being.

The recognition that some feed components might be required in greater amounts than those simply needed to prevent overt deficiency diseases suggests that the concept of essential nutrient levels needs to be reconsidered. The nutrient requirements allocated to various animal species have usually been developed based on the avoidance of deficiency diseases and the necessity for rapid growth and productivity of the animals. They have not been established based on any health maintenance or disease avoidance criteria except as mentioned above for the avoidance of deficiency diseases. Moreover nutrient requirements have only been established to cover the basic essential nutrients and there is very little information on the most useful level of various nutricines such as organic acids, antioxidants, enzymes and carotenoids. In fact the practical inclusion rate of various nutricines in animal feeds is more likely to be dictated by legislation, than by scientific requirements.

There is quite a complex relationship between dose rate of any feed component and responses in the animal as illustrated in Figure 1 (De Meulenaar, 2006) where both low or high levels of any feed component can be a source of concern. It is clearly understood that if the intake of an essential nutrient is too low deficiency symptoms will appear. At intermediate dose rates no adverse effects will be seen. Then at excessively high levels there may well be indications of undesirable effects. These could be due directly to toxic effects of the particular nutrient at high levels or also due to an imbalance in the overall diet if one nutrient is excessively high. It is also important to realize that the relationship depicted in Figure 1 is most easily observed in short term or acute studies of nutrient intakes.

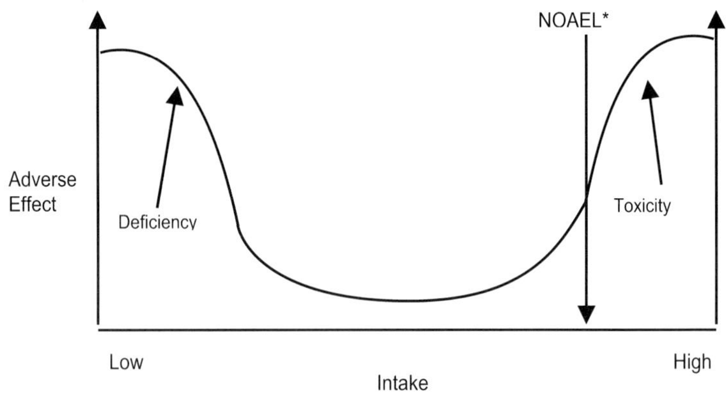

Figure 1. Generalized acute dose response for feed components, nutrients and nutricines.

*NOAEL: No observable adverse effect level

The Nutricine Concept is of interest because it raises distinctions between nutrients and nutricines in terms of essentiality and minimum or maximum dietary levels. For nutricines the same dose response as shown in Figure 1 is more difficult to observe because by definition nutricines do not readily display acute deficiency symptoms. A deficiency of various nutricines is likely to have an adverse effect upon animal health but this is more likely to be a chronic effect and therefore is not so easily demonstrated. For example a lack of the carotenoid lutein in growing chicks increases the parameters of systemic inflammation (Koutsos *et al.*, 2006). Both nutricines and nutrients will of course have upper toxic levels where adverse effects will be observed. For nutricines perhaps the most useful value would be the No Observable Adverse Effect Level (NOAEL). This is the highest dose at which no adverse effects are observed during chronic exposure. The NOAEL value is already used as the basis for determining food safety standards for humans such as the Average Daily Intake (ADI).

To develop feed formulations designed for a NbH strategy a maximium threshold level (NOAEL) of both nutrients and nutricines will need to be established rather than focussing on minimum levels. This will be the largest amount an animal can consume without an adverse effect. Once the maximum threshold levels are known it should be possible to design an effective NbH strategy which is clearly the next challenge in modern animal production. Effective nutritional recommendations should encompass the amounts of nutrients and nutricines required to optimise both growth and health of the animals.

Health assessment

On a global basis it is difficult to assess animal health yet this is becoming extremely important since animals, and particularly wild animals, are thought to be the source of more than 70% of all new emerging infectious diseases. Therefore surveillance of animals for infection with zoonotic pathogens has been proposed as one important strategy to assist in managing these infections (Kuiken *et al.*, 2005).

Health assessment of both wild animals and of animals intensively raised for food is a great task of modern nutrition. One possibility is the establishment of functional indices (Strain, 1999; Adams, 2002) in an attempt to relate nutrition to health. These functional indices can be biochemical, physiological or genetic factors which are either related to a function in target tissues or are significantly affected by changes in dietary intake of various nutricines. The optimum nutritional status may be defined in terms of the level of a food component required to avoid deficiency, to have an effect upon biomarkers or functional indicators, and prevent disease. Because many non-infectious diseases are partly caused by damage to DNA it will be important to focus attention on defining optimal requirements of key nutrients and nutricines for preventing damage to both nuclear and mitochondrial DNA (Fenech, 2002, 2003). Some nutricines such as isoflavones from soyabeans and gallate-containing polyphenols from green tea have beneficial effects in reversing gene silencing brought about by hypermethylation of DNA (Fang *et al.*, 2003, 2005).

Optimum nutrition would be achieved when a functional index reaches a certain desirable quantitative value at which it is no longer affected by dietary intake. This concept would satisfy the prevention of overt deficiency diseases, avoid toxic effects of nutrients and nutricines and maintain health. There are likely to be many dietary regimes by which adequate nutrition and consequently good health and well-being can be achieved.

A major problem in health assessment is that the relation between nutrition and health is quite different from the relation between nutrition and disease. This will require experimental designs with protocols and evaluation criteria which are different from those presently used in health research studies for drug development (Roberfroid 1999). An important aspect of NbH research is that the target population is healthy animals, and this is a very great difference from pharmaceutical research where the target population is animals with disease problems. The challenge in NbH is to design dietary modifications through intake of various nutrients and nutricines that would lead to a change in functional indices indicative of a state of good health maintenance and disease avoidance. The important function of nutrition is the ability to maintain health and avoid disease in normal animals who are ostensibly healthy.

Therefore it is necessary to develop a new concept of biomarkers for health. They need to reflect subtle changes in homeostasis and the efforts of the body (cellular system, organs and inter-organ interactions) to maintain this homeostasis. Also an appropriate biomarker preferably should include a wide variety of biological actions. Single nutrients or nutricines may have multiple known and unknown biochemical targets and physiological actions which may not be easily addressed with classical biomarkers. In addition the efficacy assessment of nutritional components is even further complicated by the fact that single dietary constituents are hardly consumed as separate entities but are part of a dietary mixture (Corthésy-Theulaz *et al.*, 2005).

There has been some progress in defining health in ageing humans (Lesourd and Mazari, 1999). Currently healthy elderly humans should have a serum albumin level of $\geq$ 39 g/l, and no deficits in Zn, Se, folic acid, and vitamins C, E, B_6 and B_{12}. Also they should not have any major acute-phase protein response with serum C-reactive protein levels being $<$30 mg/l. Such criteria have not yet been established to define animal health. Indeed major challenges that remain to be addressed are to define "normal" and "healthy" versus "unhealthy," especially in the pre-disease stage for animals raised under modern intensive conditions.

There are several global parameters of health which may well have application in the future assessment of animal health. Procedures are available to study inflammation, nucleic acid stability and status. The immune status and antioxidant status of live animals can be monitored. The composition of the microflora in the gastrointestinal tract and the fermentative capacity of the large intestine have also been considered as health assessment indices.

Inflammation

An important area for assessing the efficacy of feed ingredients in terms of health maintenance and disease avoidance is that of inflammation which leads to accelerated development of a multitude of chronic diseases. These diseases include cardiovascular problems, immune dysfunction and joint problems

There are several agents directly involved in inflammation, including cyclooxygenase-2 (COX-2), tumour necrosis factor α (TNF-α), interleukin-1 (IL-1), phospholipase A2, lipoxygenase (LOX) and inducible nitric oxide synthase (iNOS). There is a complicated pathway whereby omega-6 fatty acids such as arachidonic acid are converted by COX-2 and LOX enzymes into pro-inflammatory molecules. Down-regulation of the genes which code for the COX-2 and LOX enzymes may contribute to disease avoidance. Omega-3 fatty acids such as EPA and DHA are competitive inhibitors of COX-2 and LOX and thereby have anti-inflammatory effects. Several antioxidant nutricines such as plant phenols, vitamins, carotenoids and terpenoids have been shown to have significant beneficial effects by reducing the process of sustained inflammation.

CAROTENOIDS: In poultry there is increasing evidence that the carotenoid, lutein, plays an important role in modulating inflammation (Koutsos *et al.*, 2006). Chicks were fed a low-carotenoid diet or an enriched carotenoid diet (40 mg lutein/kg) and subjected to an inflammatory response from lipopolysaccharide. Chicks fed the low-carotenoid diet had higher body weight losses and higher plasma acute phase protein, haptoglobin, than chicks on a carotenoid enriched diet. The results suggest that a chicks without exposure to a carotenoid had increased parameters of systemic inflammation.

There is a possible correlation between the intensity of carotenoid pigmentation in avian species and health (Blount, 2004). Certain endoparasites such as coccidia can impair intestinal function in birds and therefore a superior deposition and display of carotenoids in the body might well indicate a low parasite burden and good health. Carotenoids, particularly lutein are known to be involved in immunomodulation and again good carotenoid displays may well indicate a good immune status and consequently good health.

The carotenoid concentration in the blood of avian species varies quite widely depending at least in part on the diet (Surai *et al.*, 2001). For example in laying hens the plasma carotenoid concentration was 0.7 µg/ml when fed on a standard commercial diet and increased to 3.0 µg/ml after supplementation with dietary carotenoids. The amount of carotenoids in the blood of day old chicks is influenced by the carotenoid concentration in the egg yolks. Chicks hatched from eggs laid by hens on a standard commercial diet had 3.1 µg/ml carotenoids in the plasma whereas chicks hatched form eggs enriched in carotenoids had 9.4 µg/ml. It is also interesting to note that generally much higher concentrations of carotenoids are found in the blood of wild species compared to commercial poultry. In 356 wild birds from 26 species the carotenoid concentrations varied from 0.4-74.2 μg/ml with an average of 9.4 μg/ml. It is possible that wild avian species accumulate carotenoids from the diet as part of an inherent NbH programme and therefore carotenoids concentrations in the blood might well be one index of health.

DNA damage and repair

Damage to deoxyribonucleic acids (DNA) is involved in at least two major human problems, ageing and cancer. These are not very important in the raising of animals for food, although problems of ageing are of interest in pets.

Various reactive oxygen species (ROS) and free radicals produced in cells of the animal body continually damage DNA and this must be repaired. Damage to DNA is manifested by chemical changes in the four bases, adenine, cytosine, guanine and thymine which make up the DNA molecule. Several of the oxidised molecules from DNA damage are excreted in the urine in humans in the form of nucleosides that is the base linked to the sugar deoxyribose.

The most common biomarker arises from the conversion of guanine to the nucleoside 8-hydroxy guanosine and this may be used as an index of oxidative damage to DNA. This nucleoside can measured using HPLC techniques. In a study with humans, smokers excreted 50% more 8-hydroxy-deoxyguanosine than non-smokers suggesting a 50% increase in the rate of oxidative damage to their DNA from smoking (Loft *et al.*, 1993).

Another system called "Single Cell Microgelelectrophoresise " or "COMET" assay has also been developed which involves studying the DNA in cells of animals and this can be done with blood samples (Fairbairn *et al.*, 1995). This is a more rapid technique than analysis of altered DNA bases and also reveals DNA damage due to toxic materials as well as oxidative damage. This could well have application in animal nutrition and health.

Further work in this area needs to be done on animals to see if oxidative stress can be detected in this way. Again the procedures to measure compounds such as 8-hydroxyguanosine are fairly complex and more rapid and simpler methods will be needed for widespread application in animal nutrition.

Assessment of immune status

The immune system is extremely important to protect animals against external pathogens as discussed in Chapter 6. Therefore indices of immune function should also indicate overall health status of the animal. However assessment of immune function is not an easy task and at present there is no overall simple or single measure of immunity in animals. This makes it difficult to determine the effect of a nutricine or nutrient upon the immune system. Furthermore nutritional status is unlikely to influence only one part of the immune system but will probably influence several parts of the immune system. Nevertheless several *in vitro* assays have been developed to assess the immune status.

There are two basic objectives to be achieved from assessing the immune status. The first is to determine whether a particular nutrient, nutricine, or feed formulation would improve immune function and influence immunity to infectious diseases. The second objective would be to determine whether or not the animals had developed a good immune system. The ideal scenario would be to use various indices of immunology to predict resistance to infection and to detect instances of poor immune function.

LYMPHOCYTE PROLIFERATION ASSAY: This gives information on the cell-mediated immune response. It consists of measuring the number of cells in a culture with and without the addition of a stimulatory agent or mitogen. Isolated lymphocytes are incubated with mitogens which activate division of either B- or T-lymphocytes. Various mitogens are used and some of the most common ones are: concanaviln A and phytohaemagglutin (T-cell mitogens) and lipopolysaccharide (B-cell mitogen). A decreased proliferation of the lymphocytes is usually interpreted as impaired cell-mediated immunity.

CYTOKINE PRODUCTION: Neutrophils and other cells of the immune system produce a range of protein mediators, the cytokines, such as interleukin-1 interleukin-6 and tumour necrosis factor-α. These are important in the inflammatory response which can lead to tissue damage. Cytokines are typically produced in very small amounts of picograms but procedures exist for their assay in blood.

CYTOTOXICITY ASSAY: This assay assesses the activity of cytotoxic T-lymphocytes and polymorphonuclear neutrophils that kill other cells and of NK cells that kill virus-infected and tumour cells. The release of the enzyme lactate dehydrogenase is sometimes used as an indicator of cytotocixity (Lauzon *et al,* 2005).

ACUTE PHASE PROTEINS: The acute phase proteins (APP) are a group of blood proteins which are synthesised and secreted by the liver. They increase in concentration in response to various stresses such as; inflammation of tissues, tissue injury, onset of disease or environmental stress such as transport. These various stresses generate an altered amino acid demand (Le Floc'h *et al.* 2004), which leads to the synthesis of specific APP that play crucial roles in the defence of the animal against pathogens

There are several different APP that have been identified in cattle, pigs, and poultry (Table 1) These proteins appear earlier than specific antibodies and their decrease is correlated with a reduction in the inflammatory response in mammals and poultry and therefore their concentration in the blood is an indication of health status.

Table 1. Acute phase proteins identified in various animal species.

Species	*Acute phase protein*
Cattle	Haptoglobin (Hb), Serum Amyloid A (SAA), (AGP) Albumin, Fibrinogen
Pigs	Haptoglobin, Serum Amyloid A, C-Reactive Protein (CRP) Pig Major Acute Phase Protein (Pig MAP), Albumin, Fibrinogen, α1-acid glycoprotein
Poultry	Haptoglobin, α1-acid glycoprotein, Ceruplasmin, Transferrin, Fibrinogen

Most of the APP are rich in aromatic amino acids such as; phenylalanine, tyrosine and tryptophan relative to muscle protein. (Table 2). During inflammation, APP concentrations in the blood can rise by up 100-fold. Therefore this increase in APP synthesis will require a large quantity of dietary phenylalanine, tyrosine and tryptophan.

Table 2. Amino acid composition of human acute phase and muscle proteins in g/kg.

Amino	*Protein*				
acid	*C-reactive*	*Fibrinogen*	*Haptoglobin*	*Amyloid A*	*Muscle*
Phenylalanine	105	46	30	103	40
Tyrosine	50	56	70	67	36
Tryptophan	42	35	32	45	13
Threonine	58	60	54	30	47
Lysine	71	77	92	33	98

The acute phase protein response is also associated with alterations in plasma mineral levels including the withdrawal of zinc from the blood plasma into the liver and the release of copper from tissue stores into the blood. These events are linked to growth depression and decreased production (Chamanza *et al.*, 1999).

High levels of the acute phase C-reactive protein (CRP) in the blood significantly increase the risk of cardiovascular disease in humans. There is an inverse relationship between plasma levels of CRP and total antioxidant capacity of a diet (Brighenti *et al.*, 2005). Intake of food rich in antioxidants was associated with low levels of CRP. This might be one of the mechanisms that mediate the protective effects of dietary antioxidants against chronic diseases. The total antioxidant capacity of animal feeds is not usually considered. However it might be a useful characteristic in terms of designing feeds for disease avoidance and health maintenance.

Haptoglobin is one of the major acute phase proteins in pigs and the measurement of haptoglobin levels in the blood of pigs has been proposed as a screening parameter in a health management system (Gymnich and Petersen, 2004). Haptoglobin levels correlated well with performance data. Pigs were classified into two weight-gain groups; <350 and >350 g per day. A significantly lower haptoglobin serum concentration was observed in the rearing phase with the higher daily weight gain. The systemic inflammatory response in poultry can be assessed through measuring levels of haptoglobin in the blood (Koutsos *et al.*, 2006). Chicks kept of a lutein-free diet showed increased production of haptoglobin when challenged with lipopolysaccharide from 40-175 μg/ml. Chicks fed 40 mg/kg lutein in the diet showed a reduced haptoglobin response of 120 μg/ml.

Various test kits are now available which makes it feasible to assay acute phase proteins in a routine manner to assess nutrition and health status of animals under practical conditions. For example haptoglobin concentration in bovine milk can be measured using an ELISA technique (Hiss *et al*, 2004). In cows challenged with lipopolysaccharide, to mimic a bacterial infection, there was a noticeable increase in haptoglobin after three hours. In another study haptoglobin levels in cows with mastitis reached a peak of 180 μg/ml between 24 and 48 hours after infusion with lipopolysaccharide from *Escherichia coli* (Lauzon *et al.*, 2006). These observations suggest that measurement of haptoglobin in milk might be a good diagnostic for the onset of mastitis.

Figure 2. Concentration of haptoglobin found in milk from cows infused with lipopolysaccharide to induce mastitis.

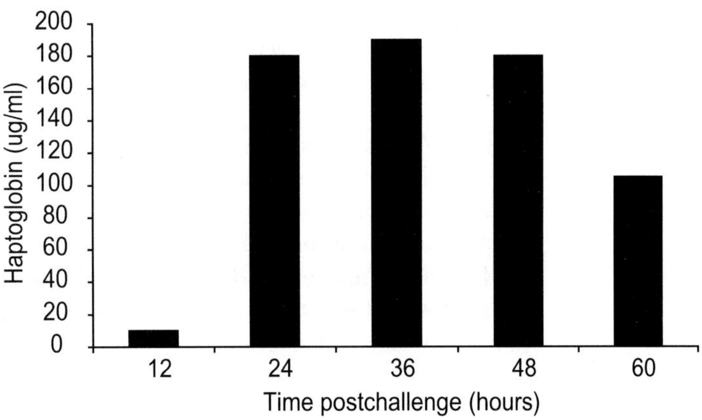

OXIDATIVE STATUS: There are two important aspects to be considered here; the oxidative status of animal feed and the oxidative status of the live animal. Animal feeds contain significant quantities of lipids, proteins and carbohydrates, all of which are susceptible to oxidation. Therefore the antioxidant capacity of a feed is an important parameter to maintain feed quality. A good oxidative status in live animals is also important in avoiding oxidative stress and the development of associated non-infectious diseases.

Animal feeds will contain varying amounts of antioxidants. These may occur from the basic feed raw materials and from antioxidants included in the feed formulation. Although the amount of exogenously added antioxidants will be known, it is practically impossible to determine the concentration of the endogenous antioxidants. Furthermore the protective effects of the antioxidant complement in a feed are derived from the combined action of the endogenous and exogenous antioxidants and from synergisms between the different antioxidant molecules. Also different antioxidants may act through different mechanisms. Therefore the total antioxidant capacity of animal feeds is an important parameter in a NbH strategy. Nevertheless it is not usually considered as it is difficult to assess because animal feeds contain many different antioxidants.

A procedure for the determination of the antioxidant capacity in feeds has been developed based on a modification of the FRAP assay combined with the DPPH assay (Smet *et al.*, 2006). The FRAP assay was originally developed to assess the antioxidant capacity of blood (Benzie and Strain, 1996). This is a relatively simple automated colorimetric test which measures the ability of blood plasma to reduce ferric ions to ferrous ions. The DPPH (2,2-diphenyl-1-picrylhydrazyl) method evaluates the neutralization of a stable radical. Using this method the combined action of the potential and concentration of the antioxidant in a feed can be determined. The total antioxidative capacity of a feed it might be a useful characteristic in terms of designing feeds for disease avoidance and health maintenance.

The FRAP assay also offers a means of assessing the antioxidant status in the blood of an animal in relation to dietary intake. For example rats fed a bilbery (*Vaccinium myrtillys* L) anthocyanin extract showed an increased antioxidant status in the blood at 3 and 6 hours after the beginning of the meal (Talavéra *et al.*, 2006). It should be possible to monitor antioxidant status in animals through the FRAP assay and this could proved useful information in a NbH programme.

MYCOTOXINS: There is always the potential for mycotoxin contamination of animal feeds to occur since moulds are ubiquitous on feed raw materials (Chapter 4). Therefore it would be useful to determine whether or not animals have been exposed to mycotoxins. A proposed biomarker to asses animal exposure to mycotoxin contaminated feeds is the increase in the ratio of sphinganine to sphingosine (SA/SO ratio) (Avantaggiato *et al.*, 2005). This biomarker is indicative of exposure of animals to the fumonisins and also of the toxic effects derived from disruption of sphingolipid metabolism in affected animals. Rats exposed to fumonisisn showed significant increases in SA/SO ratios in samples of urine and kidney but not in the liver. The use of urine samples offers a practical, non-invasive, monitoring possibility to assess the mycotoxin status of animals.

The interactive effects between several mycotoxins have been investigated using a DNA synthesis inhibition assay (Tajima *et al.* 2002). The joint action of five *Fusarium* mycotoxins, T-2 toxin, deoxynivalenol, nivalenol, zearalenone and fumonisin B_1 was studied at different dose levels. Significant synergistic actions were observed between nivalenol and T-2 toxin, deoxynivalenol and nivalenol, zearalenone and nivalenol, as well as between zearalenone and fumonisin B_1. This is not a trivial test to carry out but the concept is interesting in that it might offer the possibility to decide upon the safety of feeds from the mycotoxin point of view.

BLOOD UREA NITROGEN: This is a potential useful indicator of the efficiency of use of dietary nitrogen. This has health implications since poor utilization of feed proteins in the gastrointestinal tract provides a substrate to encourage the growth of enteric pathogens. In general a reduction in blood urea level is indicative of a more efficient use of dietary nitrogen (Owusu-Asieda *et al.*, 2003). There was strong correlation between crude protein content and blood urea level in early-weaned piglets (Nyachoti *et al.*, 2006), (Table 3). At the beginning of the experiment blood plasa urea nitrogen was between 88 and 110 mg/l. After 21 days on diets with low crude protein there was a linear response to urea nitrogen in the blood. The lowest crude protein diet gave only 32% of the blood urea nitrogen of the highest crude protein diet. It is generally accepted that reduced protein contents in pig diets give various health benefits and this might be monitored through blood urea nitrogen.

Table 3. Effect of varying crude protein content in diets of piglets on blood plasma urea nitrogen (mg/l).

Experimental	*Crude protein content of feed (%)*			
time (days)	*23*	*21*	*19*	*17*
0	110	88	88	102
7	100	82	70	58
14	95	58	50	48
21	120	62	40	38

NITRITE AND NITRATE: Nitrite and nitrate occur in blood plasma and urine and they are ultimately derived from the oxidation of nitric oxide (NO). Nitric oxide is a potent pulmonary vasodilator that can dramatically reduce the pulmonary vascular resistance and, thereby, oppose the onset of pulmonary hypertension. It has a broad spectrum of activity in both mammals and avian species and it is synthesized from arginine by the enzyme NO synthase. Nitric oxide is also produced in the body by cells such as macrophages when activated by infecting bacteria. However the NO gas molecule has a short half-life in living cells and is rapidly converted into nitrite and nitrate and excreted in the urine.

Measurement of urinary nitrite + nitrate levels has been used as a quantitative biomarker to assess total intestinal bacterial infections (Bovee-Oudenhoven *et al.*, 1997). The basic principle is that urine samples are firstly stabilised against bacterial deterioration by addition of an antibiotic to the urine samples. The nitrate in the samples is usually then chemically reduced to nitrite and the total nitrite determined by a colorimetric procedure. Automated analytical systems are available this type of approach and so it is feasible for more widespread use in assessing the status of animal health and nutrition.

In rats orally infected with *Salmonella* the levels of nitrite + nitrate increased in the urine over a six day period until it was some five-fold higher than the control rats (Bovee-Oudenhoven *et al.*, 1999). This procedure clearly has interesting applications in food animal production as infection by *Salmonella* is of major concern in terms of safe food and it might be possible to track the infection status of animals by measuring the nitrite + nitrate levels in urine samples.

Immune cells of chickens, macrophages cultured from spleen, when challenged with *Eimeria acervulina* produced increasing amounts of nitrite as the coccidiosis developed. A similar effect was seen in turkeys suffering from poult enteritis and mortality syndrome (PEMS) where again nitrite production by macrophages increased (Table 4) (Qureshi *et al.*, 1998).

Table 4. Nitrite concentration in supernatants from macrophage cultures during the progession of coccidiosis in chickens and poult enteritis and mortality syndrome (PEMS) in turkeys.

Disease	*Days post challenge*	*Nitrite (μM)*
Cocidiosis (chickens)	0	6.0
	6	21.0
PEMS (turkeys)	0	5.5
	7	20.5

Nitrite has been detected in the blood of many species, including humans, guinea pigs, minipigs, mice, monkeys, rabbits and rats (Kleinbongard *et al.*, 2003). The levels varied from 502 nmol/l in rabbits, to 191 nmol/l in rats. It appears that constitutive nitric oxide synthase activity is relatively uniform throughout the mammalian kingdom and nitrite in blood is a common characteristic

In boilers an increase in nitrite plus nitrate was detectable in the serum of broilers infused intravenously with sodium nitrite solution or injected with lipopolysaccharide (Chapman and Wideman, 2006). Both of these treatments are know to stimulate nitric oxide production. However in broilers treated with sodium nitroprusside which is an exogenous nitric oxide donor molecule any increased levels of nitric oxide were too low to be detected by standard colorimetric methods based on the nitrite assay. Possibly nitrite assay in the blood might not be sensitive enough to indicate the metabolic status of healthy animals.

LACTOBACCILLI AND COLIFORM COUNTS IN GASTROINTESTINAL TRACT: *Lactobacilli* represent a major group of micro-organisms in the small intestine and it is generally accepted that they are important to maintain good intestinal health because of their ability to control and inhibit the growth of potentially pathogenic micro-organisms such as coliforms which include various pathogenic *E. coli* strains. In piglets during the suckling period lactobacilli are dominant in the upper part of the gastrointestinal tract, due to their ability to ferment lactose from milk. After weaning however, lactobacilli numbers decrease dramatically resulting in a dilution of the inhibitory role they play in the attachment of *E. coli* to the wall of the gastrointestinal tract.

As the piglets adapt to solid feed, the microflora of the gastrointestinal tract restabilizes and the lacotobaccilli:coliform (L:C) ratio becomes more favourable for health maintenance and disease avoidance. Consequently the relative numbers of these two groups the Lactobacilli:Coliform (L:C) ratio may be considered an indicator of intestinal health.

In piglets fed varying protein levels the L:C ratio was 1.22 on day zero, falling to 1.11 on day 4 and recovered to 1.4 on days 7 and 14 (Wellock *et al.*, 2006). In this study intestinal health in the proximal colon appeared to deteriorate with increasing protein supply, with an increase in coliform numbers and a decrease in the L:C ratio. This is consistent with the concept that high protein diets provide a better environment for pathogens to develop and cause various enteric diseases.

Fermentative activity in the large intestine

As indicated in Chapter 5 fermentation in the large intestine of monogastric animals is a part of the feed digestion process and has important implications for animal health. The fermentative activity of the large intestine can be influenced by diet and this has recently been studied using a cumulative gas production system (Theodorou *et al.*, 1994). This method involves measurement of accumulating gas during fermentation. This gives a picture of the kinetics of microbial activity of the population acting as a whole. The technique has been used to study fermentative activity of the microflora from the rumen, the gastrointestinal tract of pigs and the caecae of poultry (Williams *et al.*, 2001). By using different starting substrates it is possible to study shifts in microbial populations which would be associated with the fermentation of a particular feedstuff such as resistant starch, protein or fibre. Alternatively the effect of potential nutricines in modifying fermentation patterns can be investigated.

Conclusions

Feed intake and its relationship with good animal health are important parameters since feed is usually the most expensive input in animal production. However the assessment of animal health is particularly difficult and routine procedures are not yet readily available. Feed intake is certainly influenced by health status and is a practical method to indirectly monitor animal health. Feed supply during the foetal and neonatal stages has significant implications for subsequent health and growth. Nutritional requirements still need to be refined. The general nutritional requirements established for growth and maintenance of body weight may not be equally suitable for disease avoidance, development of the immune system, and maintenance of health and well-being. There is a complex relationship between dose rate of a feed components and biological response in an animal, where both high and low levels of any component can be a source of concern. In practical nutrition the most important dose parameter is probably the NOAEL (No Observable Adverse Effect Level). Health assessment of growing animals is a major challenge for modern nutrition because the relation between nutrition and health is quite different from that between nutrition and disease. There are several global parameters of health which may well have application in the future assessment of animal health. Measurement of inflammation and in particular the influence of carotenoids on inflammation is important. DNA stability and repair can be assessed. The immune status can be monitored.through various assays such as cytokine and acute phase protein production. Techniques are available to study the oxidative status of feed and of live animals. Urea, nitrite and nitrate in blood are also useful indices of health status. The composition of the microflora in the gastrointestinal tract and the fermentative capacity of the large intestine also provide information on animal health.

References

Adams, C. A. (2002). TOTAL NUTRITION Feeding Animals for Health and Growth, Nottingham University Press, Nottingham UK, 244 pp.

Avantaggiato, G., Solfrizzo, M. and Visconti, A. (2005). Recent advances on the use of adsorbent materials for detoxification of *Fusarium* mycotoxins. Food Additives and Contaminants, 22: 379-388.

Benzie, I. F. F. and Strain, J. J. (1996). The ferric reducing ability of plasma (FRAP) as a measure of "antioxidant power": The FRAP assay. Analytical Biochemistry, 239: 70-76.

Bovee-Oudenhoven, I. M. J., Termont, D. S. M. L., Weerkamp, A. H., Faassen-Peters, M. A. W. and Van der Meer, R. (1997). Dietary calcium inhibits intestinal colonization and translocation of salmonella in rats. Gastroenterology, 113: 550-557.

Bovee-Oudenhoven, I. M., Wissink, M. L., Wouters, J. T. and Van der Meer, R. (1999). Dietary calcium phosphate stimulates intestinal lactobacilli and decreases the severity of a salmonella infection in rats. Journal of Nutrition, 129: 607-612.

Blount, J. D. (2004). Carotenoids and life-history evolution in animals. Archives of Biochemistry and Biophysics, 430: 10-15.

Brighenti, F., Valtueña, S., Pellegrini, N., Ardirò, D., Del Rio, D., Salvatore, S., Piatti, P-M., Serafini, M. and Zavaroni, I. (2005). Total antioxidant capacity of the diet is inversely and independently related to plasma concentration of high-sensitivity C-reactive protein in adult Italian subjects. British Journal of Nutrition, 93: 619-625.

Chamanza, R., van Veen, L., Tivapasi, M. T. and Toussaint, M. J. M. (1999). Acute phase proteins in the domestic fowl. World's Poultry Science Journal, 55:61-71.

Chapman, M. E. and Wideman, Jr., R. F. (2006). Evaluation of total plasma nitric oxide concentrations in broilers infused intravenously with sodium nitrite, lipopolysaccharide, aminoguanidine, and sodium nitroprusside. Poultry Science, 85: 312-320.

Corthésy-Theulaz, I., den Dunnen, J. T., Ferré, P., Geurts, J. M. W., Müller, M., van Belzen, N. and van Ommen, B. (2005). Nutrigenomics: The impact of biomics technology on nutrition research. Annals of Nutrition and Metabolism, 49: 355-365.

De Meulenaar, B. (2006). Chemical hazards. In:*Safety in the agri-food chain* eds: P. A. Luning, F. Devlieghere and R. Verhé. Wageningen Academic Publishers, Netherlands pp.145-208

Fairbairn, D. W., Olive, P.L., and O'Neill, K. L. (1995). The Comet Assay: A comprehensive review. Mutation Research, 339: 37-59.

Fang, M.Z., Wang, Y., Ai, N., Hou, Z., Sun, Y., Lu, H., Welsh, W. and Yang C. S. (2003). Tea polyphenol (-)-epigallocatechin-3-gallate inhibits DNA methyltransferase and reactivates methylation-silenced genes in cancer cell lines. Cancer Research, 63: 7563-7570.

Fang, M.Z., Chen, D., Sun, Y., Jin, Z., Christman, J. K. and Yang C. S. (2005). Reversal of hypermethylation and reactivation of $p16^{INK4a}$,

*RAR*b, and *MGMT* genes by genistein and other isoflavones from soy. Clinical Cancer Research, 11: 7033-7041.

Fenech, M. (2002). Micronutrient and genomic stability : a new paradigm for recommended dietary allowances (RDAs). Food and Chemical Toxicology, 40: 1113-1117.

Fenech, M. (2003). Nutritional treatment of genome instability: a paradigm shift in disease prevention and in the setting of recommended dietary allowances. Nutrition Research Reviews, 16: 109-122.

Gous, R. M. (2006). Predicting nutrient responses in poultry: future challenges. Proceedings of the British Society of Animal Science p.216.

Gymnich, S. and Petersen, B. (2004). Haptoglobin as a screening parameter in health management systems in piglet rearing. Pig News and Information, 23: 111N-118N.

Hiss, S., Mielenz, M., Bruckmaier, R. M. and Sauerwein, H. (2004). Haptoglobin concentrations in blood and milk after endotoxin challenge and quantification of mammary Hp mRNA expression. Journal of Dairy Science, 87: 3778-3784.

Kleinbongard, P., Dejam, A., Lauer, T., Rassaf, T., Schindler, A., Picker, O., Scheeren, T., Gödecke, A., Schrader, J., Schulz, R., Heusch, G., Schaub, G. A., Bryan, N. S., Feelisch, M. and Kelm, M. (2003). Plasma nitrite reflects constitutive nitric oxide synthase activity in mammals. Free Radical Biology and Medicine, 35: 790-796.

Koutsos, E. A., López, J. C. G. and Klasing, K. C. (2006). Carotenoids from in ovo or dietary sources blunt systemic indices of the inflammatory response in growing chicks (*Gallus gallus domesticus*). Journal of Nutrition, 136: 1027-1031.

Kuiken, T., Leighton, F. A., Fouchier, R. A. M., LeDuc, J. W., Peiris, J. S. M., Schudel, A., Stöhr, K. and Osterhaus, A. D. M. E. (2005). Pathogen surveillance in animals. Science, 309: 1680-1681.

Langley-Evans, S. C (*editor*) (2004). Experimental models of hypertension and cardiovascular disease. *In* Fetal nutrition and adult disease: Programming of chronic disease through fetal exposure to undernutrition. pp. 129-156. Wallingford, Oxon, CABI.

Langley-Evans, S. C. (2006). Developmental programming of health and disease. Proceedings of the Nutrition Society, 65: 97-105.

Lauzon, K., Zhao, X., Bouetard, A., Delbecchi, L., Paquette, B. and Lacasse, P. (2005). Antioxidants to prevent bovine neutrophil-induced mammary epithelial cell damage. Journal of Dairy Science, 88: 4295-4303.

Lauzon, K., Zhao, X., and Lacasse, P. (2006). Deferoxamine reduces tissue damage during endotoxin-induced mastitis in dairy cows. Journal of Dairy Science, 89: 3846-3857

Le Floc'h, N., Melchior, D. and Obled, C. (2004). Modification of protein and amino acid metabolism during inflammation and immune system activation. Livestock Production Science, 87: 37-45.

Lesourd, B. and Mazari, L. (1999). Nutrition and immunity in the elderly.

Proceedings of the Nutrition Society, 58: 685-695.

Loft, S., Fischer-Nielsen, A. and Jeding I. B. (1993). 8-Hydroxyguanosine as a urinary marker of oxidative DNA damage. Journal of Toxicology and Environmental Health, 40: 391-404.

Lucas, A. (1991). Programming by early nutrition in man. Ciba Foundation Symposium, 156: 38-50.

Nyachoti, C. M., Omogbenigum, F. O., Rademacher, M. and Blank, G. (2006). Performance responses and indicators of gastrointestinal health in early-weaned piglest fed low-protein amino acid-supplemented diets. Journal of Animal Science, 84: 125-134.

Owusu-Asiedu, A., Nyachoti, C. M., Baidoo, S. K., Marquardt, R. R. and Yang, X. (2003). Response of early-weaned pigs to an enterotoxigenic Escherichia coli (K88) challenge when fed diets containing spray dried porcine plasma or pea protein isolate plus egg yolk antibodies. Journal of Animal Science, 81: 1781-1789.

Qureshi, M. A., Hussain, I. and Heggen, C. L. (1998). Understanding immunology in disease development and control. Poultry Science, 77: 1126-1129.

Roberfroid, M. B. (1999). Concepts in functional food: the case of inulin and oligofructose. Journal of Nutrition, 129 (Suppl.) 1398S-1401S.

Sandberg, F. B., Emmans, G. C. and Kyriazakis, I. (2006). A model for predicting feed intake of growing animals during exposure to pathogens. Journal of Animal Science, 84: 1552-1566.

Smet, K., Raes, K. and de Smet, S. (2006). Novel approaches in measuring the antioxidative potential of animal feeds: the FRAP and DPPH methods. Journal of the Science of Food and Agriculture, 86: 2412-2416.

Strain, J. J. (1999). Optimal nutrition: an overview. Proceedings of the Nutrition Society, 395-396.

Surai, P. F., Speake, B. K., and Sparks, N. H. C. (2001). Carotenoids in avian nutrition and embryonic development. 1. Absorption, availability, and levels in plasma and yolk. Journal of Poultry Science, 38: 1-27.

Tajima O., Schoen, E. D., Feron, V. J. and Groten J. P. (2002). Statistically designed experiments in a tiered approach to screen mixtures of *Fusarium* mycotoxins for possible interactions. Food and Chemical Toxicology, 40: 685-695.

Talavéra, S., Felgines, C., Texier, O., Besson, C., Mazur, A., Lamaison, J-L. and Rémésy, C. (2006). Bioavaiability of a bilberry anthocyanin extract and its impact on plasma antioxidant capacity in rats. Journal of the Science of Food and Agriculture, 86: 90-97.

Theodorou, M. K., Williams, B. A., Dhanoa, M. S., McAllan, A. B. and France, J. (1994). A simple gas production method using a pressure transducer to determine fermentation kinetics of ruminant feeds. Animal Feed Science and Technology, 48: 185-197.

Wellock, I. J., Fortomaris, P. D., Houdijk, J. G. M. and Kyriazakis, I. (2006). The effect of dietary protein supply on the performance and risk of post-weaning enteric disorders in newly weaned pigs. Animal Science, 82: 327-335.

Williams, B. A., Verstegen, M. W. A. and Tamminga, S. (2001). Fermentation in the large intestine of single-stomached animals and its relationship to animal health. Nutrition Research Reviews, 14: 207-227.

9 General Conclusions

Good animal health is an important parameter for the efficient production of the large volumes of food of animal origin which are currently required, and the even greater volumes which will be required in the future. Animal health has a great impact not only upon the security of an important food supply, but it also has impacts upon human health and upon international trade and economics. Consequently health maintenance and disease avoidance in the animals raised for food in modern animal production is a major global challenge.

Threats to animal health come in many forms. The environment is a perennial threat and source of infectious disease and good hygiene is obviously important here. The quality of drinking water is crucial to good animal health. Feeds are frequently contaminated with fungi, mycotoxins and bacteria and the hygiene status of feeds is also an important parameter. Both the water and the feed supplies must be considered as potential disease vectors. The necessity to raise large numbers of animals in relatively small areas also subjects these animals to considerable stress during the raising period. This will be manifested as increased susceptibility to infectious diseases and the development of many non-infectious diseases.

It is clear that the major route to maintain health and avoid disease must be through nutrition since therapeutic treatment of unhealthy animals is neither a desirable nor in many cases a practical solution. Therefore Nutrition-based Health (NbH) will become an important strategy in animal production. It will be important to demonstrate to the consumer that the mechanisms of modern animal production pay suitable attention to the health of the animals as well as to their growth and productivity. An NbH strategy also responds to consumer and legislative concerns where the link between diet and health is increasingly under investigation. There is considerable interest and attention nowadays directed towards an NbH approach both for humans and for animals.

Animal feeds and human foods however, are extremely complex containing both nutrients and bioactive components, the nutricines, and a NbH approach must utilize both groups of ingredients. In animal nutrition feed exerts both an external effect inside the gastrointestinal tract and an internal effect upon metabolism of the animal body.

The balance between good health or disease comes from an interaction between the genetic make-up or the genome of the animal and the environment in which it is raised. This gives the phenotype. Nutrition may be considered as one environmental factor that has many ramifications. It affects genomic stability which is a fundamental cause of disease. Many dietary compounds influence the expression sequence of genotype into phenotype. Feed ingredients may directly affect gene expression or they may act through the activation of transcription factor systems that regulate specific sets of genes in different tissues and under different environmental conditions. The relationship between nutrition and expression of the genotype, or nutrigenomics, has important practical implications. It is an attempt to provide a genetic and molecular understanding for how common dietary chemicals, particularly nutricines, affect the balance between health and disease. This in turn would lead to an improvement in the understanding of the impact of nutrition on health, and could guide nutritional programmes.

The integrity of the gastrointestinal tract is a major health determinant as enteric diseases cause serious problems and economic losses in animal production. The normal healthly gastrointestinal tract develops a very extensive microflora which contributes to protection against pathogens and also ferments undigested feed components in the large intestine. Fermentation products, particularly butyric acid, are valuable nutrients for the enterocytes in the large intestine. Several amino acids such as arginine, glutamine, threonine and histidine help to maintain the integrity of the gastrointestinal tract.

Enteric diseases arise when pathogenic microorganisms invade the gastrointestinal tract and there is an important diet-pathogen interaction in mitigating enteric diseases. A basic objective in the development of NbH must be to identify and to exploit various feed raw materials and other bioactive feed ingredients, nutricines, that can inhibit pathogen adhesion, inhibit pathogen growth and ensure that the diet does not increase the virulence of pathogens. Feed formulation can play a useful role in managing enteric disease.

Some anti-adhesion factors have been identified such as non-digestible oligosaccharides and tannins. Reduced protein content and the use of cooked rice in piglet diets have given some benefits. Nutricines such as organic acids, enzymes, non-digestible oligosaccharides and essential oils are able to modify the microflora in the gastrointestinal tract with positive health benefits. Feed also influences pathogen virulence, particularly necrotic enteritis in poultry. Good antioxidant status in feeds is beneficial in reducing the pathogenicity of some viruses. Iron status influence the susceptibility of animals to infectious diseases and iron chelators such as deferoxamine or organic acids may play a useful role here.

The health status of animals is frequently challenged by mycotoxin contamination of feed raw materials and feeds. Mycotoxins pose a double threat to animal production, as direct toxins and also as immunosuppressors which will increase, the susceptibility of animals to infectious diseases. Management and control of mycotoxins is technically well-established and precautions can be taken at time of harvest and during the storage of raw materials to reduce or avoid mould contamination. Mycotoxin binding products can be incorporated into feeds to reduce the absorption of mycotoxins from the gastrointestinal tract. Various dietary interventions can be utilized to minimise the effect of mycotoxins on animal growth and health.

It is clear that in modern animal production the support of an efficient immune system is extremely important to protect animal health. In particular the innate immune response is critical to disease avoidance in animals since it is a very rapid defence mechanism. It is well accepted that nutrition influences the robustness of the immune system but it is still not clear how the various nutrients and nutricines specifically affect the immune system. It is not established whether or not dietary requirements for growth are adequate to support the immune system. Lutein is a good example here where it has little effect upon growth but plays an important role in supporting the immune system. Various non-digestible oligosaccharides also have immunomodulating effects. Increasing the ratio of *n*-3 to *n*-6 PUFA in feeds gives benefits in terms of supporting the immune system.

Another important and continuous threat to animal health comes from the Oxygen Paradox. Animals must use oxygen for metabolism yet oxygen is also deleterious to animal health and well-being. During normal metabolism there is always the production of reactive oxygen species (ROS) and reactive nitrogen species (RNS). These are kept under control by a range of antioxidant enzymes and antioxidant molecules in the body. An oxidative stress develops when ROS and RNS accumulate and overwhelm the endogenous antioxidant protection mechanisms in the body. This may in turn lead to the development of a wide range of both non-infectious and infectious disease syndromes. Nutrition has a major influence upon the pro-oxidant/antioxidant balance in the body and there are numerous potential antioxidant nutricines in feeds. Oxidative stress has serious effects upon animal health and can cause increased DNA damage, affect foetal development, induce neurotoxicity and increase the susceptibility to mastitis. There are several important non-infectious diseases in animals; hypertension, ascites, mastitis, retention of foetal membranes, lung problems, calcium status, and bone and joint problems, which are influenced by oxidative stress. Oxidative stress also plays a role in the onset of some infectious diseases, particularly those of viral origin and antioxidant status of the animals may be important here. Antioxidant nutricines are certainly important components of an NbH strategy as they influence so many factors related to health.

Feed intake and its relationship with good animal health are important parameters since feed is usually the most expensive input in animal production. However the assessment of animal health is particularly difficult and routine procedures are not yet readily available. Moreover the general nutritional requirements established for growth and maintenance of body weight may not be equally suitable for disease avoidance, development of the immune system, and maintenance of health and well-being. There is a complex relationship between the dose rate of feed components and the biological responses in an animal, where both high and low levels of any component can be a source of concern. In practical nutrition the most important dose parameter is probably the NOAEL (No Observable Adverse Effect Level).

Health assessment of growing animals is a major challenge for modern nutrition because the relation between nutrition and health is quite different from that between nutrition and disease. Measurement of inflammation and in particular the influence of carotenoids on inflammation is important. DNA stability and repair can be assessed. The immune status can be monitored through various assays such as cytokine and acute phase protein production. Techniques are available to study the oxidative status of feed and of live animals and antioxidant status of live animals. Urea, nitrite and nitrate in blood are also useful indices of health status. The composition of the microflora in the gastrointestinal tract and the fermentative capacity of the large intestine also provide information on animal health.

There is clearly much more research needed to fully understand the relationship between nutrition and health. This is a topic of major concern for both animal and human health and a Nutrition-based Health (NbH) strategy must be applied in the production of animals for food.

INDEX